Pathway to Diagnosis and Management of Toothaches

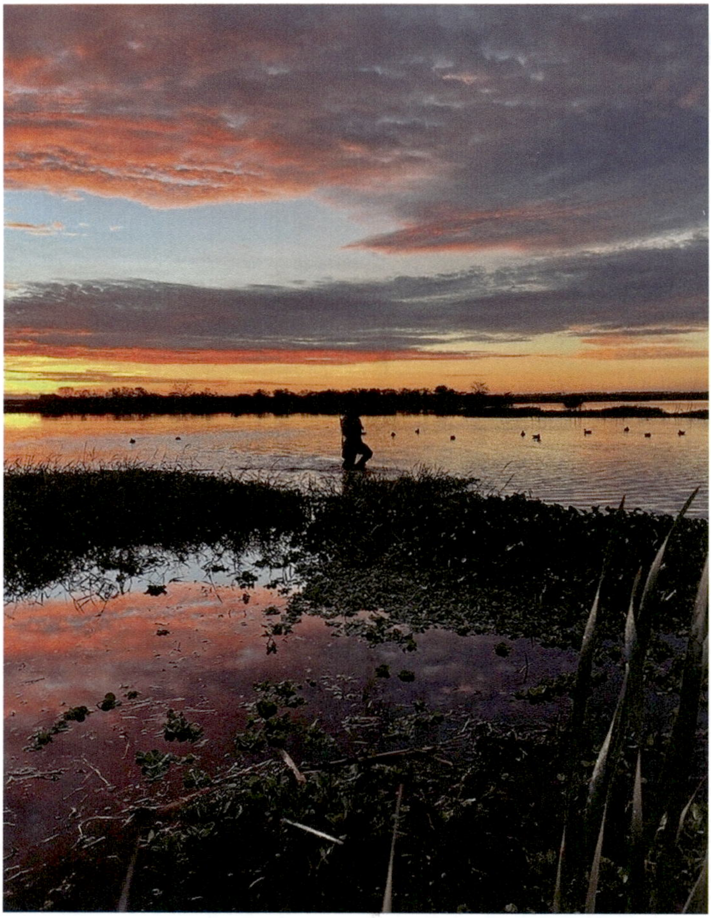

The cover picture was taken by Dr. John Hardeman on Nov. 28, 2021, at 6:48 am near Cocoa, FL, while hunting with my son. It was selected to remind the reader that arriving at a final diagnosis is not a simple path but requires adjustment in direction based on information gained along the journey. Just as slogging through a swamp requires processing information gained with each step before advancing to the next, the diagnostic process requires adjustments based on information gained rather than a predetermined process applied to every situation. Dr. Hardeman is the former chairman of the UFCD-OMFS and an amateur photographer.

Ernest Lado • Robert Caudle

Pathway to Diagnosis and Management of Toothaches

A General Dentist's Perspective

Springer

Ernest Lado
Department of Oral and Maxillofacial Surgery
University of Florida, College of Dentistry
Gainesville, FL, USA

Robert Caudle
Department of Oral and Maxillofacial Surgery
University of Florida, College of Dentistry
Gainesville, FL, USA

ISBN 978-3-031-75261-2 ISBN 978-3-031-75262-9 (eBook)
https://doi.org/10.1007/978-3-031-75262-9

This Springer imprint is published by the registered company Springer Nature Switzerland AG
The registered company address is: Gewerbestrasse 11, 6330 Cham, Switzerland

This work is dedicated to the thousands of dentists I have had the privilege of instructing over the past half century. I enjoyed private practice but cherish my years of continued scholarship that afforded me an opportunity to share my acquired knowledge with subsequent generations.

Foreword

In this book, *Pathway to Diagnosis and Management of Toothaches*, Dr. Ernie Lado shares 57 years of experience, knowledge, and wisdom about the physiologic and psychologic aspects of toothache pain. He practiced for more than a decade as a general dentist where he gained first-hand experience on the quandaries of dental pain. For the remaining 40+ years, Dr. Lado has shared these experiences with student dentists as they matriculated their way through the process of understanding dental pain. He has authored many notebooks and guides on the topic for the students but has never shared his expertise with the general dental audience. Now he has summarized his knowledge and wisdom in this treatise and presents it from the perspective of a general dentist.

He has attempted in every way to include the physiologic processes of dental pain and has provided a straightforward approach to reaching an accurate dental diagnosis. This book is an abridged guide to the clinical examination and diagnosis of dental pain. It focuses on the role that pain plays in identifying the source of the chief complaint, thereby reducing erroneous findings or flawed interpretation of diagnostic tests. Readers will find guidance on the collection of data, performance of clinical exams, and assessment of pain associated with specific components of the dental complex. Special emphasis is placed upon the condition of the pulp, starting with the normal pulp and progressing through the partially necrotic pulp and ultimately to pulp necrosis. Information is provided on a preferred method of conducting and interpreting diagnostic tests, as well as diagnosis and prognosis of fractured teeth. The final portion of this book is dedicated to periodontal pain. This section discusses the normal and inflamed periodontium, radicular periodontitis, apical periodontitis, and the endo-perio diagnosis. This book will serve as a reference for all dentists, as the diagnosis of toothaches is a daily process in practice. It can be a complicated process since the present pedagogues fail to address the intricacies involved in the precise etiology of clinical signs and symptoms.

Gainesville, FL, USA John H. Hardeman

Preface

How many times have you heard, "The dentist pulled the wrong tooth?" Unfortunately, there is some truth to the statement. <Pubmed.gov> lists hundreds of publications on phantom tooth pain caused by primary lesions or dysfunction of the peripheral or central nervous system, including trigeminal neuralgia, atypical odontalgia, traumatic neuropathies, postherpetic neuropathies [1], angina, and among others. Any of them can lead to an inaccurate diagnosis, resulting in unwarranted, irreversible treatments, including endodontic and/or surgical procedures. When a patient presents with a "toothache," they often point to what they believe to be the offender. To expedite treatment, we (dentists) are sometimes inclined to accept the patient's insistence that a particular tooth is the problem and proceed with treatment without a thorough evaluation and a confirmed diagnosis.

In 2009 and updated in 2013, the American Association of Endodontists (AAE) proposed new diagnostic terminology to "facilitate communication between dentists." This terminology is based mainly on the interpretation of past and present symptoms and diagnostic test results, with a casual consideration of the biophysiological process causing the problem. Once "diagnostic" findings fit a preponderance of symptoms comprising an AAE diagnosis, this author (EL) observes an inclination to settle on a "diagnosis" with minimal thought given to the underlying cause. The working diagnosis may be a product of an analysis of flawed information provided by the patient and skewed diagnostic tests. Unfortunately, the methods of diagnostic testing and interpretation are not standard and may account for a number of specious diagnoses.

An internet search for publications supporting the reliability and reproducibility of the new AAE's diagnoses nomenclature is sparse. In fact, the nomenclature was adopted by a committee, in which several members opposed its acceptance. An online survey found "minority reports suggest that there was still greater than 25% of the respondents who did not follow consensus," while consensus was determined to be 51% of the responders [2]. The online survey results "suggest an awareness for the specialty to develop better diagnostic tools and terminology that are biologically, and metric-based.[1]"

[1] Core idea in metric-based learning a subfield of machine learning where algorithms are applied to meta-data. Weng, Lilian (30 November 2018)." Open AI Blog. Retrieved 27 October 2019.

As late as 2020, an editorial appeared in the *International Endodontic Journal*, calling for a review of diagnostic nomenclature and terminology used by endodontists in which the authors "believe that there is an overwhelming need for a review of the existing nomenclature (*proposed by the AAE*) related to pulp and periapical diagnostics" and, rather than basing diagnosis on ad hoc clinical finding, "Pain should be considered as a core parameter [3]."

This work focuses on a coherent approach to conduct and interpret diagnostic tests and align the results with subjective findings, so as to consider the bio-physiologic process leading to the patients' existent chief complaint. This approach demands "critical thinking," a process frequently touted but often unheeded.

This process includes consideration of the two major sensory nerve fibers that dominate transmission of dental pain: a-∂ fibers, located mainly in the coronal portion of the dental pulp, with extensions accompanying odontoblastic processes in the dentinal tubules, transmit a "sharp shooting" pain, while C-fibers, mainly found deeper in the pulp and periodontium, transmit a "dull, aching" pain.

It is said that if you want to catch a criminal, "follow the money." My adaption to the saying is "if you want to identify the source of a toothache, follow cell lysis and production of PgE_2."

You will notice this work accentuates a repetition of the role *of* PgE_2 and the specific sensory fibers that conduct dental pain. This is done purposefully to etch the concept that *pain is a product of injured or dying cells* and encourage you (the diagnostician) to consider bio-physiologies' role in causing dental pain, rather than simply relying on patients' subjective reports of pain and their reactions to unfettered diagnostic tests into a diagnostic schema to arrive at a diagnosis.

A review of *Pathway to Diagnosis and Management of Toothaches* will improve your understanding of the basis by which dental pain arises, the role of specific sensory nerves, and how this information applies to diagnosis and ultimately treatment. If the information presented here in is assimilated and thoughtfully applied, the incidence of misdiagnoses should diminish.

When I was in private general practice (over 40 years ago), dentistry was considered as much an Art as a Science. Today, dentistry has morphed more into a science than an art but still leaves room for growth. My objective in writing this book is to foster your curiosity in the science of dentistry, thereby contributing to your professional advancement. My appreciation for research peaked while assembling information for this book. I found the existing information available via the Internet provides a wealth of knowledge, fulfilling the axiom "life-long learning." I suggest you find a topic of interest and investigate it on the world wide web. You may be astonished by what you find.

References

1. Feller L, Khammissa RAG, Fourie J, Bouckaert M, Lemmer J. Postherpetic neuralgia and trigeminal neuralgia. Pain Res Treat. 2017;2017:1681765. https://doi.org/10.1155/2017/1681765. Epub 2017 Dec 5. PMID: 29359044; PMCID: PMC5735631.

2. Glickman GN, Bakland LK, Fouad AF, Hargreaves KM, Schwartz SA. Diagnostic terminology: report of an online survey. J Endod. 2009;35(12):1625–33. https://doi.org/10.1016/j.joen.2009.09.034.
3. Rechenberg DK, Zehnder M. Call for a review of diagnostic nomenclature and terminology used in Endodontics. Int Endod J. 2020;53(10):1315–17. https://doi.org/10.1111/iej.13374.

Gainesville, FL, USA Ernest Lado
Gainesville, FL, USA Robert Caudle

The original version of the book has been revised. A correction to this book can be found at https://doi.org/10.1007/978-3-031-75262-9_7

Acknowledgments

Tooth Illustrations:

The illustrations of teeth depicting the progression of tooth pain were created by Gregg Stewart, DMD, the first student I had the privilege of mentoring. His comment follows. The rigors of dental school, and the exacting nature of our profession requires an energy outlet to relax, recharge and refresh our minds. I found that in art.

The saying, "A picture is worth a thousand words," never rang truer than the moment I started learning about dental pain. Many texts offered detailed descriptions of the types of pain, but visualization of that pain was absent. Under Dr. Lado's guidance, I was able to utilize my artistic abilities and create the "pictures" of different types of pain. The intention was to instantly capture the "where" and "why" of dental pain. My hope is that these images will help others in diagnosing and understanding dental-related pain.

Contents

About the Author

Ernest Lado is a general dentist who graduated from Georgetown University College of Dentistry in 1967 and practiced general dentistry for 13 years, of which ten were spent in solo private practice. Dr. Lado was appointed in 1981, as an instructor in the Department of Oral Medicine, College of Dentistry, University of Florida. He was promoted to Assistant Professor in 1983 and promoted to Associate Professor in 1988. Shortly after, Dr. Lado was transferred to oral maxillofacial surgery, where he was assigned to the Student Oral Surgery Clinic. He presently oversees students in diagnosing, extracting, and referring patients to other specific specialties for definitive treatment. Over the past 56 years, Dr. Lado has assessed tens of thousands of toothaches and has witnessed numerous misdiagnoses. He has also taught treatment planning, radiology, and emergency preparedness for the dental office and oversaw the urgent care clinic. Dr. Lado initiated the UF Sterilization Monitoring Service in 1989 and monitored both in-house and private practice sterilizers for over 10 years before the college disbanded the service to accommodate needed space for research.

Robert M. Caudle is a Professor at the University of Florida. He graduated from Humboldt State University in 1981 and received his Ph.D. from the University of Illinois at Chicago in 1988. Dr. Caudle's research examines the mechanisms of pain transmission and the molecular changes in the peripheral and central nervous systems that lead to chronic pain. He has published over 90 papers and teaches courses on pain mechanisms and pain management to dental, medical, and graduate students.

Tooth Pain

1

1.1 Introduction

Dental pain is nature's way of alerting a patient to an assault on the dental complex and the primary motive patients seek dental care [1]. There have been efforts to introduce clinically relevant terminology that labels specific diagnoses of "toothaches." Some historic "terminologies" were based on histologic findings while others were based on clinical signs and symptoms. The histologic approach was not widely accepted in part because it did not allow for a definitive diagnosis prior to microscopic examination of the pulp, while some diagnostic terminologies based on existent clinical signs and symptoms fail to identify the underlying cause of the reported pain [2, 3].

A contemporary classification introduced by the American Association of Endodontists (AAE) in 2009 and modified in 2013 identifies "snapshots" of static odontogenic "diagnoses" based mainly on existent signs and symptoms. The stated purpose for this classification is to facilitate communication between endodontists, dentists, and researchers as well as to direct proper treatment [4]. Unfortunately, this classification does not foster an in-depth understanding as to the basis for dental pain and may lead to a specious diagnosis. AAE's taxonomy bases a "diagnosis" on subjective pain from the pulp and dental complex with little consideration given to the bio-physiologic process resulting in pain.

This work encourages the inclusion of bio-physiological processes involved in causing "toothaches" rather than relying simply on subjective symptoms and objective test results directing the diagnosis. Odontogenic pain may arise from any of the components of the dental complex or combinations thereof and must be adequately diagnosed in order to determine appropriate treatment.

When cells die their membranes are lysed, releasing arachidonic acid that is converted to prostaglandin E_2 (PgE_2) by cyclooxygenase [5–7]. Recent bio-physiologic studies show a high correlation of inflammatory mediators (especially PgE_2) lowering the pain threshold of specific nerve fibers populating defined parts

E. Lado, R. Caudle, *Pathway to Diagnosis and Management of Toothaches*,
https://doi.org/10.1007/978-3-031-75262-9_1

of the dental complex. *By identifying characteristics of reported pain, one may be directed to the specific part or parts of the complex that is under attack.*

Pain heralds something is awry, and patients often seek prompt relief by resorting to OTC palliative remedies. These remedies may provide some relief but can mask diagnostic test results leading to a specious diagnosis. It is essential to question the patient as to their effort to seek temporary relief with OTC remedies (including systemic and topical analgesics) so as not to nullify the diagnostic findings.

Test results must be timely, but the diagnosis should also corroborate the history of past symptoms (Anamnesis). With the introduction of AAE's classification I (EL) have noticed a tendency to diagnose odontogenic pain based on existent symptoms and test results along with a failure to consider symptomatic changes that have transpired from the onset of the problem. There should be an attempt to confirm the diagnosis is consistent with the history as well as existent symptoms and not just the result of coincidental supportive findings.

NOTE: "*Non-odontogenic toothaches are often difficult to identify and can challenge the diagnostic ability of the clinician. The most important step toward proper management of toothaches is to be suspicious that the reported problem may not be of dental origin*" [8].

"Radiating pain" to the temporal region should cause one to suspect a condition involving the maxillary premolars or molars. However, if the patient complains of an earache, "referred" pain from mandibular teeth (more frequently than not, a molar) should be considered.

NOTE: *Radiating pain extends directly from the affected area to its surroundings while referred pain arises in a location away from the affected area,*

Keep in mind toothaches often involve more than one element of the dental complex. Hence, the entire complex should be considered when evaluating a problem.

1.2 Innervation of Dental Complex

As previously stated, pain is a distress signal alerting that something is awry (cells dying). The following discussion introduces the predominant sensory nerves found in the dental complex. Transmission of specific characteristics of pain is nerve specific, so one can deduce the specific part or parts of the complex involved.

The main nerves found in pulp are the a-∂, a-β, and C-fibers. A-β fibers represent a low percentage (7%) of A-fibers, are similar to a-∂ fibers, and play a minor role in pain. A-∂ fibers are myelinated fibers that have a fast conduction speed and a low stimulation threshold. They are found mainly in the coronal portion of the pulp with some accompanying odontoblastic processes into the dentinal tubules and transmit a sharp, short duration pain. They may be considered the sentry's that alert the dental complex to an assault.

According to Brännström, pain is provoked by hydrodynamic changes within the dental tubule, caused by drilling, acidic foods, cold air, touch, and changes in osmotic pressure, which can lead to rapid fluid movement within the tubules, stimulating the mechanosensitive nerve endings to transmit a short, sharp initial pain.

This warning may be sufficient for the pulp to respond by stimulating formation of reparative dentin and hopefully for the patient to seek professional evaluation and treatment. Brännström's hydrodynamic theory seems to apply mainly to exposed dentin that is not protected with enamel [9]. An exception may be pain provoked by procedures employing caustic agents such as bleaching of enamel [10].

A-∂ fibers are highly oxygen dependent; consequently, if the circulation within the pulp is compromised, the a-∂ fibers degrade and an aching pain characteristic of transmission from C-fibers becomes dominant [11].

C-fibers are unmyelinated slow conducting, sensory nerves with smaller diameter but higher stimulation thresholds than a-∂ fibers and are found deeper in the pulp. Once they transmit pain spontaneously and continuously, the health status of the pulp should be considered "irreversible." That leaves two options for resolution, root canal treatment (RCT) or extraction (EXT).

The typical clinical symptoms of an irreversible pulpitis (involving the C-fibers) without apical involvement present as a constant, elusive, aching, sometimes throbbing, pain, that is difficult to locate. It may be aggravated by heat and sometimes is provoked following exposure to cold (i.e., ice cream). This is analogous to a condition identified in World War I known as "Tooth Squeeze" also referred to as "Aerodontalgia" or "Barodontalgia" where the degraded pulp leaves a void (trapped air) within the confines of the sealed chamber and temperature changes affect the pressure of the trapped air.

1.3 Odontogenic Pain

A confounding condition occurs when the a-∂ fibers lose the ability to function because they are highly oxygen dependent. However, C-fibers continue to function longer than A-fibers because they are less dependent on oxygen [11]. "The location of the C-fibers deeper within the nerve bundles may account for the aching pain from the vital but diseased pulp." It is important to recognize that dental pulp lacks proprioceptive fibers, and the patient may have difficulty locating the precise tooth causing the pain. We often tap on teeth to locate the problem but unless the periodontium is involved, the percussion test will be uninformative. Fortunately, the periodontium is replete with proprioceptive fibers so once inflammatory mediators reach the apex, localization of the offending tooth is readily discernable [12].

Challenges to the odontoblastic processes (residing in dentinal tubules) cause a short duration, sharp painful response from the a-∂ fibers found accompanying the processes, hopefully prompting a visit to the dentist for evaluation and treatment. If the assault is ongoing but not lethal to the odontoblast, a protective layer of dentin may form, and the sensitivity should wane. If on the other hand, the tubules remain opened to the oral environment the odontoblasts degrade, providing direct access to the pulp chamber. In effect, leaving a micro-exposure to viable pulp [13].

As the assault continues, a pronounced inflammatory reaction occurs at the pulp-dentin junction ending with apoptosis of the odontoblasts and formation of PgE_2 resulting in dentinal hypersensitivity (DH), an exaggerated response from a normally painful stimulus. This is not to be confused with normal dentinal sensitivity (DS) since exposed viable dentin is expected to transmit a short duration sharp pain.

For the sake of simplicity, "dentinal sensitivity" (DS) designates a "Normal" response of exposed dentin to an outside stimulus, while "dental hypersensitivity" (DH) designates an exaggerated response from a normally painful stimulus.

The question arises WHY?

Why should Brännström's hydrodynamic theory be the cause of both DS and DH?

It has been shown that dentinal tubules associated with the crown are smaller and "S" shaped and the tubules found below the DEJ are bigger and straighter. With this in mind, "fluid shifts across dentin are thought to cause sufficient shear forces on odontoblasts, nerve endings, nearby fibroblasts, and blood vessels". "provide diffusion channels for noxious (i.e., bacterial products) substances which diffuse inward toward the pulp, where they can activate the immune system, provide chemotactic stimuli, cytokine production, and produce pain and pulpal inflammation" [14]. I (EL) perceive this to be the defining condition between DS and DH. I base this on the observation that DH seems to occur most often along the exposed root (where the tubules are larger and straighter) and rarely from coronal dentin, protected by enamel and tubules are smaller and S shaped, making it more difficult for bacteria to negotiate their way to the pulp.

Let's review the bio-physiology of dental pain, again! As mentioned previously, the predominant sensory nerves associated with teeth and their supportive structures are the a-∂, a-β, and C-fibers. When stimulated, the a-∂ fibers (found mainly in the coronal part of the pulp and associated with odontoblasts and processes found in dentin) transmit sharp pain while the C-fibers (found deeper in the canal) transmit an aching pain. C-fibers are also the predominant sensory nerves found in the periodontium. The sensory threshold of these nerves is lowered in the presence of pain mediators, particularly prostaglandin E_2 (PgE_2) that is produced from arachidonic acid released from ruptured cell membranes. As more cells are lysed, more PgE_2 is produced. The higher the concentration of PgE_2, the lower the pain threshold, ultimately resulting in spontaneous pain [6]. This sequence is a key paradigm to a biophysiologic approach to diagnosis of dental pain.

NOTE: *As I stated in the Preface, "If you want to find the source of a toothache...follow the* PgE_2*."*

As cell membranes are lysed, arachidonic acid is released and acted on by cyclooxygenase, producing PgE_2. As more cells are attacked and membranes are disrupted, levels of PgE_2 increase, and permeate viable tissue, lowering the pain threshold of sensory nerves, initiating symptoms of a "*reversible pulpitis*." These symptoms usually manifest as a sharp intense pain of short duration and should quickly disappear once the challenge is removed without lingering aching pain. On the other hand, if the pulp fails to heal and cells continue to degrade, more PgE_2 permeates the deeper portion of the pulp where C-fibers predominate. The initial sharp pain caused by stimulation of the a-∂ fibers wanes and a spontaneous aching pain transmitted by the C-fibers prevails. Once spontaneous aching pain occurs and there is a past history of pain (as suggested by Dr. Bender—next paragraph), the ability of the pulp to repair itself is presumed lost and is termed "*Irreversible Pulpitis*." Up until recently, it was presumed that teeth experiencing spontaneous pain without a prior history of pain was sufficient to declare it "reversible" and to delay root canal treatment (RCT) rather, attempt a pulp cap if the tooth structure was sound enough to support a restoration.

Evidence gathered by Dr. Bender "points to the fact that the incidence of pain increases as the histopathosis (sic) worsens. On interrogation, patients who manifest severe or referred pain almost always give a previous history of pain in the tooth with the ache. Eighty percent of patients who report a previous history of pain manifest histopathologic evidence of chronic partial pulpitis with partial necrosis, the untreatable category, for which endodontics or extraction is indicated. The other 20% exhibit histopathosis of the pulp with slight inflammation to chronic partial pulpitis without necrosis, a treatable category." "Clinically, one can determine the degree of pulp histopathosis by asking the patient about a previous history of pain in the involved tooth." "This history of previous pain adds another dimension in diagnosis for the clinician as to whether the painful pulpitis is reversible" [15].

I find the assumption that "…one can determine the degree of pulp histopathosis by asking the patient about a previous history of pain…" perplexing; especially when considering AAE's taxonomy that states: "**Asymptomatic Irreversible Pulpitis** is a clinical diagnosis based on subjective and objective findings indicating that the vital inflamed pulp is incapable of healing, and that root canal treatment is indicated. These cases have no clinical symptoms and usually respond normally to thermal testing but may have had trauma or deep caries that would likely result in exposure following removal."[1]

Huh? I think this needs resolution!

It is my presumption the first pain involves the sensibility of a-∂ fibers and is discussed earlier noting that the A-fibers were the sentry alerting an attack on the tooth. They signal the pulp to muster a defense by initiating an inflammatory reaction along with substance P and CGRP lowering the pain thresholds of the sensory nerves. In effect the patient is being warned to get help as soon as possible. Failure to seek evaluation and treatment results in the violation of the defensive wall established by reparative dentin and the inflammatory response. This violation constitutes the "First" pain (reversible pulpitis) patients experience prior to the diagnosis "irreversible."

Once the defense breaks down, bacteria have access to vital pulp tissue and along with their toxins, destroy cells, lysing the cell membranes, releasing arachidonic acid that in turn is acted upon by cyclooxygenase producing (YOU GUESSED IT) Prostaglandin E_2. PgE_2 begins to permeate the pulp, moving apically, lowering the sensory threshold of C-fibers, and giving rise to a spontaneous, continuous aching pain.

This aching pain may throb especially when the patient lies down. Throbbing/aching pain has been proposed to result from the effects of pulse pressure (the

[1] https://www.aae.org/specialty/wp-content/uploads/sites/2/2017/07/endodonticdiagnosisfall2013.pdf.

pressure differential between systolic and diastolic blood pressure) on contents confined within the rigid pulp canal. As the patients' head is brought to the same level or lower than the heart, the pulse pressure within the pulp chamber increases, intensifying the pain (See "pressure wave" page 17).

Parenthetically, an extended exposure to cold may temporarily relieve the pain just as ice reduces pain from cell injury and may account for some questionable outcomes of thermal diagnostic tests and clinical symptoms.

If timely treatment is sought and the initial attack is stopped, the inflamed pulp lays down reparative dentin, the sensitivity wanes, and the pulp returns to normal.

1.4 Non-odontogenic Pain

NOTE: *"Non-odontogenic toothaches are often difficult to identify and can challenge the diagnostic ability of the clinician. An important step toward proper management of toothaches is to suspect that the reported problem may not be of dental origin"* [8]. *On the other hand, radiating or referred pain may be diverting attention from an odontogenic origin. Example follows.*

"Radiating pain" to the temporal region should cause one to suspect a condition involving the maxillary premolars or molars. If the patient complains of an earache, "referred" pain from mandibular teeth (more frequently than not, a molar) should be considered.

NOTE: *Radiating pain extends directly from the affected area to its immediate surroundings while referred pain arises in a location away from the affected area.*

Keep in mind toothaches often involve more than one element of the dental complex. Hence, the entire complex must be considered when evaluating a problem.

Recognizing, cell death (apoptosis) results in the production of PgE_2, should it arise from an inflamed sinus, the sensory threshold of the nerves supplying the neighboring maxillary molars and premolars may also experience increased sensitivity to masticatory and thermal challenges without an inflammatory response within the pulp. This is an example of radiating pain from the sinus inflammation causing the pulp to respond as if it were inflamed.

The absence of contributing findings (i.e., large restoration, extensive caries, periodontal problems, etc.) that would suggest an assault on the pulp or trauma to the dental complex should direct you to consider the possibility of a non-odontogenic etiology and attention should be focused on other potential causes such as sinusitis, or referred pain to the lower jaw from a heart problem. Pain from an inflamed sinus can be misinterpreted as a "*Symptomatic Irreversible Pulpitis*" (SIP) caused by an inflamed pulp and/or a "*Symptomatic Apical Periodontitis*" (SAP) due to the increased levels of PgE_2. A pulpal origin must be ruled out as the cause. The key here is to interrogate the patient about the history of the pain as well as allergies and overall health and examine both teeth and sinus. Of course, parafunctional habits such as bruxing/clenching must be ruled out as well as a history of spontaneous pulp pain that was relieved by using an over-the-counter (OTC) toothache remedy containing eugenol or benzocaine. Obviously, a radiographic image would be helpful.

NOTE: A pulpitis should be suspected if there is, a sedative dressing, history of a pulp cap, etching acid placed on dentin, improperly cured composite restoration, failure to place a non-caustic base or other evidence of a previous violation of the pulp should all be considered.

1.5 Diagnosis of Dental Pain

Before examining how each component of the dental complex contributes to tooth pain, it is important that we speak the same language. Pain has a language all its own and is made clear by Melzack and Torgerson in "On the *Language of Pain*" [16]. A review of this publication is highly recommended. A table of pain descriptors is included in the Addendum (Chap. 6).

It is important to be clear when describing pain attributed to a toothache. Confusion often arises when words are misused. For instance, the word "Sharp" is often used instead of "Severe" to express the intensity of pain. "Sharp" is used to describe the quality of pain, while "Severe" should be reserved to express intensity of pain. Inappropriate use of words can lead one to a flawed conclusion. The following discussion will help clarify communication as it relates to the diagnosis of toothaches.

Diagnosis of Dental Pain Involves Three Cognitive Procedures

A. Anamnesis (History of Chief Complaint from initial symptoms to present)
B. Clinical Exam (signs/symptoms, visual inspection, and diagnostic tests)
C. Assessment (Assignment of pain to specific components of the dental complex.)

1.5.1 Anamnesis

Simply stated, this is the history of the chief complaint from its' onset as reported by the patient, to the existent status. Envisioning the progression of the symptoms, from its' start should lead to a final diagnosis. When assessing the information consider that the health status of the pulp and types of nerves stimulated account for the differences in characteristics of pain [17, 18],

1. Inception and clinical course
2. Onset and aggravating or relieving factors
3. Characteristics of pain (see page 8 "Four Characteristics of Pain")

1.5.1.1 Inception and Clinical Course

Establish when the pain started and how it has changed over time. Keep in mind certain sensory nerve fibers prevail in specific tissues and transmit specific types (quality) of pain (i.e., "Sharp Shooting" vs "Dull Aching"). This allows one to track the progression of the condition and the dental complex involved. A patient reporting a prior history of spontaneous aching pain without a history of a sharp component suggests a periodontal problem, whereas a patient presenting with a constant aching pain, but recalls a period of sharp pain to thermal challenges, suggests the progression of pulpal-periapical problem. The status of the pulp and the types of nerves stimulated explain the differences in characteristics of pain. Describing the changes in symptoms over time should facilitate diagnosis.

1.5.1.2 Onset

Onset of pain may be described as either spontaneous, elicited (provoked) or both. Spontaneous pain occurs in the absence of stimulating factors, whereas elicited pain is provoked by thermal, postural, chemical, osmotic, barometric, etc., changes. Elicited pulp pain w/o a history of spontaneous pain suggests a pulp capable of self-repair once the irritant is removed. This is considered as "Reversible Pulpitis." On the other hand, spontaneous pulpal pain suggests the pulp is no longer capable of self-repair and is considered as "Irreversible Pulpitis" [19].

1.5.1.3 Characteristics of Pain

There are four characteristics applicable to dental pain (pattern, quality, intensity, distribution). It is important to recognize the meaning of words commonly used to describe each character and to appreciate the distinction between them. Unfortunately, as previously mentioned, improper use or misinterpretation of descriptive words can lead to the wrong diagnosis. A common example is the word "Dull" (assigned to "*quality*" of pain) is sometimes used to mean "Mild" (assigned to "*intensity*" of pain). The quality of pain is attributed to specific sensory nerve fibers discussed. It is important to use the proper descriptive term so that the pain associated with the chief complaint is attributed to specific nerve types leading to the source of the pain. (See Table of Descriptors)

Four Characteristics of Pain Are as Follows

Intensity of pain is subjective and prone to misinterpretation. This in itself can lead to misdiagnosis. Therefore, it is necessary to understand the four major characteristics of pain that accompanies toothaches.

1. ***Pattern*:** describes the temporal nature of pain. It may be continuous or intermittent (transient). Continuous or prolonged pain is described as not "letting up" while transient pain comes and goes. An example of a continuous pain is an aching muscle, while a muscle spasm is an intermittent (transient) pain. It is common for the pattern of pain to change over time.

   A patient may complain of a tooth becoming increasingly sensitive to percussion and *palpation* with an underlying pattern of continuous aching pain of moderate to severe intensity but elicits a severe sharp pain when challenged by a thermal stimulus. Pulp pain may change to a pulsating or throbbing ache, eventually returning to the constant aching pain that existed prior to the thermal challenge. This scenario would <u>not</u> be suggestive of a tooth with a completely necrotic pulp but may be seen with a partial pulp necrosis. As the discussion of causes of tooth pain continues, you will begin to appreciate the mechanisms controlling pain and follow the path to its origin.

NOTE: Pain upon palpation of the vestibular areas at the level of the tooth apex suggests an apical abscess, even in an absence of swelling. The levels of PgE_2 increase significantly with an apical abscess (infection) as opposed to an apical periodontitis (inflammation). The pain threshold of attendant sensory nerves decreases as levels of PgE_2 increase due to the degradation of proximate cell membranes.

A multirooted tooth with an inflamed pulp may exhibit both severe sharp "shooting" pain and/or an aching pain when the pain threshold of a-∂ and C-fibers is lowered by PgE_2, and the tooth is not sensitive to percussion/palpation. This finding is consistent with a "Symptomatic Irreversible Pulpitis" w/o apical involvement. If the tooth is also sensitive to biting or percussion, but not sensitive to palpation, then there is an attendant inflammatory reaction. However, should the tooth become sensitive to palpation an infection exists and an abscess is forming at the apex. If the tooth is fractured and the fracture extends to the periodontium, pain will be evident upon palpation at the level of the fracture, not at the level of the apex. Pain from the fracture results from tissue injury and not an infection. This conundrum is explained by the proximity of the fracture to the surface mucosa as opposed to the apical inflammation found deeper in bone (see Chap. 3 on Fractured teeth.)

Sensitivity to palpation at the level of the apex results from an overwhelming production of PgE_2 due to degradation of the attendant cell that occurs with an abscess. A single-rooted tooth is not likely to respond similarly to a multirooted tooth since an apical abscess precludes vitality of the pulp in a single-rooted tooth. Exception should be noted for a partially necrotic pulp or "Barodontalgia," to be discussed later.

2. ***Quality***: refers to the type of pain the patient is experiencing, its' dullness (aching) or brightness (sharpness).

   NOTE: *Quality is not to be confused with the "intensity" of spontaneous pain.*

   Elicited *sharp pain* is characteristic of dental sensitivity and coronal pulpal pain arising from a-∂ fibers, whereas spontaneous *aching pain* arises from the C-fibers found in the deeper portion of the pulp or the periodontium. The type of sensory nerves being stimulated determines the quality of pain. A-∂ nerve fibers, located in the coronal portion of the pulp, transmit sharp pain whereas C-fibers, found deeper in the pulp chamber and supportive periodontium, transmit an aching pain. A word of caution here! Although the sharp lancinating pain caused by stimulation of the a-∂ fibers may be quite intense, it does not account for the prolonged lingering aching pain that follows a thermal challenge. The prolonged aching pain (following the sharp pain caused by the thermal challenge to a-∂ fibers) arises from stimulation of the C-fibers located deeper within the canal. Since it may be presumed that cellular degradation usually starts within the pulp chamber, the pain mediators (especially PgE_2) spread apically, lowering the pain threshold of the deeper C-fibers resulting in a spontaneous prolonged aching pain. This is pathognomonic of an "Irreversible Pulpitis."

3. ***Intensity:*** Dental pain may be divided into 3 levels of intensity (mild, moderate, and severe). **Mild** pain may be described as annoying but not distressing and the

patient can function normally. **Moderate** pain may be described as distressing but can be controlled with over-the-counter analgesics, allowing the patient to function normally. **Severe** pain prevents normal functioning despite using a strong analgesic. An example of severe pain is a patient's ability to chew is impaired due to the pain even after taking a strong analgesic. The intensity of pain is relative to the level of PgE_2 produced and the remaining viable sensory nerves. Three levels of pain can be perceived in terms of "thresholds" (see discussion in Addendum).

Mild: Threshold of Sensation: annoying but can function normally.

Moderate: Threshold of Pain: hurts but can be controlled with over-the-counter (OTC) analgesics.

Severe: Threshold of Tolerance: hurts so much function is impaired, and pain cannot be managed with analgesics. Radiates to surrounding areas.

4. ***Distribution:*** Pain may be localized or diffuse (widespread). The ability to localize pain facilitates identifying the source of the toothache. Frequently, however; pain will "radiate" to the surrounding proximal area. "Referred pain," on the other hand, will appear to arise from an area away from the source. For instance, pain from the maxillary posterior teeth will often radiate to the temporal regions whereas pain from a heart attack may be referred to the lower jaw or left arm. Referred tooth pain will often originate from the opposing ipsilateral arch (top to bottom or bottom to top) never to or from the opposite side [20]

Application: The information obtained in the history should include the following:

Inception and Clinical Course

When did it first start?	How has it changed over time?

Onset

Elicited	Spontaneous

Characteristics

Intensity	Quality	Pattern	Distribution
Mild/bothersome **Moderate/**hurts **Severe/**can't stand it anymore	**Sharp/**lancinating shooting, stabbing **Dull/**aching, deep, boring, gnawing	**Continuous/**constant **Pulsing/**throbbing **Intermittent/**comes and goes	**Localized** vs **Diffuse** **Radiating** vs **Referred**

Upon completion of the anamnesis, you should have a reasonable idea as to the cause of the chief complaint. A review of the "Language of Pain"[2] and recognizing

[2] See Melzack and Torgerson in "*On the Language of Pain*".

the role of the major pain receptors will, together, improve your diagnostic skills and ultimately in communication with colleges.

1.5.2 Clinical Exam

Signs/symptoms, visual inspection percussion, palpation are basic elements leading to a diagnosis. The use of a mouth mirror and explorer, coupled with a thorough clinical history often provides sufficient information to arrive at an accurate diagnosis.

However, should this not be the case, further information must be obtained with radiographic imaging, periodontal probing, and diagnostic tests. Selective tests should be conducted so as to reproduce existent symptoms. Reproduction of reported symptoms validates the offending tooth has been correctly identified. Do not rely on a single test when additional tests are needed to confirm or rule out other possibilities. For instance, sensitivity to percussion may lead one to suspect an inflamed pulp but it is not pathognomonic. But, as has been mentioned, percussion could be a sign of a number of odontogenic (i.e., Bruxism) and non-odontogenic (i.e., Sinusitis) disorders (see "Diagnostic Tests" Chap. 4).

Once the chief complaint has been established, the reported pain may be categorized into one of the major categories (Pulpal, Periodontal, Both, or Other). Pain may also be categorized based on the *intensity*. (Mild, Moderate, Severe) as well as *quality* (Sharp vs Aching) as termed by the patient. As previously mentioned, sharp pain (especially to thermal challenges) customarily arises from the dentin and coronal pulp tissue enervated mainly with a-∂ fibers, whereas aching pain is most often associated with the radicular pulp and periodontium that is mainly enervated by C-fibers.

Objective signs must be consistent with the subjective symptoms reported by the patient. *Diagnostic tests should be selected to confirm reported existent symptoms in order to assure that the offending tooth has in fact been identified.*

In the case of a suspected pulpitis, one must establish the "Onset" of pain; that is, whether the pain is spontaneous, elicited or both. The presence of spontaneous aching pain from the pulp is suggestive of an irreversible pulpitis whereas elicited sharp pain alone is characteristic of a dentinal sensitivity (DS), or dentinal hypersensitivity (DH) a reversible pulpitis, cracked tooth or pain of non-odontogenic origin, i.e., trigeminal neuralgia.

NOTE: *The following 2 paradigms apply only to pulpal pain and not to be confused with periodontal pain.*

$$\text{Tooth pain} \xrightarrow{\underline{\text{Elicited}}\ \text{Sharp Pain}-\text{short duration}} \begin{matrix} \text{Normal Pulp} \\ \text{or} \\ \text{Reversible Pulpitis} \end{matrix}$$

As inflammatory mediators progress apically and C-fibers are affected, the elicited sharp pain wanes and is overridden by a prolonged aching pain.

$$\text{Toothache} \xrightarrow{\substack{\text{Elicited sharp pain followed by a spontaneous}\\ \text{and or prolonged aching pain}}} \text{Irreversible Pulpitis}$$

Appropriate pulp tests are thermal, dentinal sensitivity, and electric pulp testing (EPT) and in very rare instances, a test cavity preparation in the case of full coverage. The odds are that extensive caries will be found under a crown upon access to tooth structure and restorability should be determined once the crown is removed.

Other methods of pulp testing are available to evaluate the tooth's vascular supply such as a Laser Doppler Flowmeter (LDF) or pulse oximetry but are expensive and impactable for clinic use [21].

A non-pulpal periodontal condition may be suspected if the patient presents with spontaneous aching pain without a history of sharp pain, or trauma. It can be further categorized by its' location on the root, that is: marginal, radicular, or periapical.

$$\text{Toothache?} \xrightarrow[\substack{\text{Possible pulp pain if the pulp involves an accessory canal, a fracture,}\\ \text{DS/DH (exposed dentin) or a compromised blood supply to the pulp.}}]{\underline{\text{Spontaneous}}\text{ aching pain}} \text{Periodontitis}\left\{\begin{array}{l}\text{Marginal}\\ \text{Radicular}\\ \text{Periapical}\end{array}\right.$$

Marginal periodontal conditions, such as gingivitis and periodontitis, are most frequently diagnosed upon visual examination and periodontal probing. Tender, swollen gingiva that bleeds upon gentle probing are cardinal signs of periodontal problems. Fetor and punched out papilla suggest an acute necrotizing ulcerative gingivitis (ANUG).

Radicular periodontal conditions are most frequently identified by periodontal probing, palpation, and radiographs. Periapical lesions are readily identified by apical percussion, palpation, and radiographic imaging (PARL).

"PARL" is an anacronym used in radiology applied to a periapical radiolucency prior to identifying symptoms associated with the lesion. Once symptoms are determined, a diagnostic label is appropriate.

NOTE: *Pulpal-periapical pathosis will invariably elicit a history of signs or symptoms consistent with both the associated pulpal condition, as well as the periodontium.*

A periodontal condition may cause a dentinal hypersensitivity (DH) from exposed dentin or pulpitis originating from an accessory canal. Pain from DH may fade with time as the tubule is mineralized. However, involvement of an accessory canal may allow bacteria access to the pulp canal resulting in an infected pulp that advances on to an *irreversible pulpitis* and eventually pulp necrosis. So, it is very possible to have an elicited "Sharp" pulpal pain after periodontal debridement in the absence of caries. Appropriate tests include visual inspection, dentinal sensitivity, thermal, electric pulp test (EPT), palpation, percussion, mobility, periodontal probing, radiographic imaging, or any combination thereof that is deemed necessary.

Classifying odontogenic pain as to its origin (pulp vs periodontium) can be challenging and requires confirmation based on properly conducted tests and assessment of the findings. Once the chief complaint is established to be of pulpal origin, a diagnosis may be made in accordance with the recent AAE diagnostic taxonomy.

Decisions to provide endodontic treatment must be based on an overall treatment plan, remaining bone support, the patient's wishes, and financial considerations.

It should be noted that radiographic examination is very helpful in confirming the diagnosis of many of these conditions; however, the absence of pathologic radiographic findings alone is not conclusive. For example, the apex of a fenestrated root can appear normal upon radiographic imaging despite the presence of a fluctuant apical abscess in the vestibule. Also, bone loss from a beginning apical abscess may take days to appear radiographically in spite of the apical area being painful to palpation.

1.5.3 Assessment

Assessment (Assignment of pain to specific dental components). Each component of the dental complex is discussed separately thus there will be frequent repetition. My apologies, but I think it is important to maintain context when considering how each component is affected.

1.5.3.1 Enamel

Since enamel is mainly inorganic (96% Hydroxyapatite) and lacks a nerve supply, it is not a direct source of dental pain. However, teeth with micro-fractures (crazing) in the enamel may respond with pain to non-noxious challenges including thermal and chewing forces, but the response should be short-lived and not spontaneous [22]. This is consistent with Brännström's hydrodynamic theory for dentinal pain.

The reason for this pain is that micro-fractures in enamel expose the underlying dentinal tubules at the dentin-enamel complex. These tubules house odontogenic processes accompanied by a-∂ nerve fibers. *Repeated stimulation of these fibers is believed to result in an Allodynia (an exaggerated painful response to repetitive non-noxious stimuli.*) [23, 24] As previously mentioned, Brännström's hydrodynamic theory accounts for fluid distortion within the dentinal tubule as well as the odontoblast processes [9]. It is reasonable to accept this distortion could be sufficient to activate neural transmission from the a-∂ fibers accompanying the process, resulting dental sensitivity (DS). However, several theories as to the etiology of dental hypersensitivity (DH) are reviewed in the (Addendum (DH) Chap. 6).

Once the tubules desiccate, the integrity of the cell membrane is disrupted releasing arachidonic acid that is in turn acted on by cyclooxygenase contributing to the production of prostaglandins. This increase in PgE_2 lowers the pain threshold of the a-∂ fibers resulting in dentinal hypersensitivity (DH) to thermal stimuli as well as tactile forces. Inflammatory mediators rush to the site and a full-blown inflammatory reaction begins. More on this in the section on Dentin.

Patients presenting with crazed or fractured enamel often complain of intense pain that is easily mistaken for pulpitis. Given time, repeated challenges ideally stimulate the formation of reparative dentin, walling off the dentinal tubules, and symptoms wane. However, a failure of odontoblasts to lay down reparative dentin and wall-off these tubules can result in accentuated elicited pain (DH).

Noxious chemicals that penetrate enamel and reach dentin, such as those used in bleaching and etching procedures, caustic chemicals (acids) found in improperly cured bonding restorations and even acidic foods (citrus) can provoke an allodynia by repeated exposure of the sensory apparatus located in the dentinal tubules [25, 26]. Other chemicals including some found in whitening and tarter-control toothpastes can also trigger an allodynia [27, 28]. Tarter-control toothpastes rely on chelating chemicals that dissolve the calcified calculus. It also dissolves the minerals that seal the dental tubule subjecting its' contents to the oral environment.

There are several types of allodynia as follows [29]:

1. **Tactile Allodynia** (also known as *mechanical* allodynia)
   Static Mechanical Allodynia: Pain to touch. (Pain upon biting and/or percussion w/o infection)
   Dynamic Mechanical Allodynia: Pain resulting from repeated light stroking or rubbing.
2. **Thermal Allodynia**: Pain triggered by Δ temperature that normally is not painful. (Dentinal hypersensitivity)
3. **Movement Allodynia**: Pain triggered by normal movement of joints and muscles. (TMJ)

If the odontoblasts underlying the affected tubules remain viable reparative dentin will form, and the sensitivity will fade in time (~3 months possibly longer). Fluoride gels and other desensitizing agents (such as GLUMA® desensitizer) may protect the odontoblastic processes by sealing the outer part of the dentinal tubules, preventing noxious chemicals from penetrating the pulp [30].

When crazed enamel is suspected as the cause of pain, the health of the pulp should be re-evaluated in 2–3 weeks to rule out pulpitis. If the tooth remains hypersensitive to non-noxious challenges for 3 months or more, it is likely the odontoblasts have been rendered incapable of laying down secondary or reparative dentin and undifferentiated mesenchymal cells are not going to transform into odontoblastic type cells as might be anticipated in young patients with open apexes. Pulp-capping would not be a viable option. Although the painful response from a non-noxious stimulus may not be spontaneous (i.e., does not meet the criteria for "*irreversible pulpitis*"), the patient may find the recurring discomfort so intolerable they elect endodontic treatment followed by full coverage or extraction just to be rid the pain. With time it is conceivable that the pulp will undergo a quiet death (asymptomatic irreversible pulpitis (AIP) and eventual necrosis).

***NOTE**: Contrary to AAE's definition of AIP this tooth has clinical symptoms and does not respond normally to thermal challenges. It does not, however, demonstrate spontaneous pain as would be expected from an irreversible pulpitis.*

1.5.3.2 Dentin

Recall dentin is about 35% organic and the rest 65% mineral (hydroxyapatite). The organic portion (odontoblastic processes and nerve fibers found within the dentinal tubules) is responsible for sensory perception. Stimulation of the a-∂ afferent nerve fibers transmit a short duration sharp pain characteristic of dentinal sensitivity [31].

Pain attributed to dentinal sensitivity (DS) is a normal, physiologic response (hydrodynamic theory of dental pain) in a healthy, non-inflamed dental pulp. It has been suggested that dentinal hypersensitivity (DH) results from a failure to eliminate the irritant causing allodynia. On the other hand, acids from bacterial plaque, acidic foods, and other chelating agents may dissolve mineral deposits thus opening the sealed dental tubules, allowing bacteria and other toxins to readily penetrate the tubules, provoking repetitive challenges to the odontoblastic processes along with the accompanying a-∂ nerve fibers, ultimately lysing the odontoblastic processes, releasing arachidonic acid that is then converted to PgE_2 [32, 33]. This heralds the onset of a "*reversible pulpitis*" characterized by sharp pain that quickly fades once the irritant is removed. Keep in mind that unless mineral salts accumulate to seal the open dentinal tubules, tertiary dentin is laid down, or the dentin is sealed with a restoration, the patent tubules provide direct access to the pulp from the oral environment through which noxious agents and bacteria can enter and provoke an inflammatory response.

A challenge to freshly exposed dentinal tubules normally provokes an intense sharp pain (DS) that should disappear shortly after the challenge is removed. This includes recent Class II fractures involving enamel and dentin (not including the pulp) or simply from exposed dentin due to abrasion, attrition, abfraction or erosion, or simply a lost restoration.

Pain caused by stimulation of a-∂ nerve fibers within the dentinal tubules should disappear moments after the challenge is removed unless noxious irritants (i.e., citric acid) invade the pulp or an allodynia sets in. If the assault destroys odontoblasts but does not overwhelm the healing capacity of the pulp in teeth with open apexes, undifferentiated mesenchymal cells within the younger pulp can differentiate into odontoblast-like cells that will in turn produce tertiary (reparative) dentin at the site of attack [34]. This transition of mesenchymal cells is possible mainly in a well vascularized pulp of a recently erupted tooth but is rare in mature patients with restricted apexes and pulps with diminished blood supply.

The newly formed layer of protective dentin not only retards the progression of decay, but also blocks bacteria, their metabolites, and other noxious irritants from entering the pulp through the open dentinal tubules, hence protecting the pulp at least temporarily. Sensitivity should wane once the odontogenic processes are destroyed, and tertiary dentin has formed.

Failure of the pain to disappear (or it becomes spontaneous) indicates further cell lysis increasing the level of inflammatory mediators, especially PgE_2 and eventually the condition will progress on to an "*Irreversible Pulpitis*." On the other hand, the pulp may undergo apoptosis, leaving a void in the pulp canal that at some point may be infected through the process known as anachoresis. (Circulating bacteria enter a void and colonize where they are protected from immune response.)

As the bacteria and their toxins penetrate through the dentin to the pulp, they will trigger more cellular death and a whole new set of symptoms arise as you will see from the discussion of the next component of the dental complex: "Pulp."

1.5.3.3 Pulp

The pulp provides a number of functions that help maintain the integrity of the tooth. It may be divided into two sections: coronal and radicular. The center of the coronal pulp and radicular region supply nutrients and help maintain the health of the pulp. The peripheral region of the coronal pulp (including the odontoblastic processes and a-∂ nerve fibers) is responsible for warning of an eminent threat with pain and protects the pulp from foreign attacks by stimulating the production of reparative dentin.

The pulp has four defined functions including [35]:

- ***Formative***: Odontoblasts produce primary dentin as the tooth forms and protects the pulpal tissue.
- ***Nutritive***: The pulp keeps the organic components of the surrounding mineralized tissue supplied with moisture and nutrients. Reduces tendency of the dentin (root) to become brittle.
- ***Protective/Sensory***: Extremes in temperature, pressure, or trauma to the dentin or pulp are perceived as pain. (Alarm system warning of impending harm to tooth)
- ***Defensive/Reparative***: By odontoblasts (and when available, mesenchymal cells that transform into odontoblastic-like cells) capable of forming reparative or tertiary dentin will further protect the viable pulp tissue from assault.

As mentioned, the major types of afferent nerve fibers found in the pulp that mediate the sensation of pain are the myelinated a-∂ nerve fibers and unmyelinated C-fibers.

The a-∂ fibers are preferentially located in the periphery of the coronal pulp where they are in close association with the odontoblasts and dentinal tubules. C-fibers typically terminate in the pulp proper either as free nerve endings or as branches that surround blood vessels.

Recall, stimulation of a-∂ fibers provoke a sharp, shooting pain, whereas stimulation of the C-fibers provokes a longer lasting, aching pain. Given the type of pain associated with these afferent sensory fibers, one can surmise the extent of pulp involvement [36].

NOTE: *The pulp does not have proprioceptive fibers therefore patients may have difficulty locating the offending tooth unless the periodontium (where proprioceptive fibers are found) is also involved* [37].

Since pulpal pain signals an assault on the pulp proper, when addressing a patients' pain, it is important to first identify the responsible tooth and then assess the capacity of the pulp to heal. The assessment weighs heavily on the onset of pulpal pain (i.e., spontaneous aching pulpal pain is suggestive of an irreversible pulpitis, whereas elicited pulpal pain (in the absence of spontaneous aching pain) is suggestive of a reversible pulpitis.)

If pulpitis is suspected, locating the offending tooth may be best accomplished by thermal testing. But if inflammatory mediators have spread to the apex (where proprioceptive fibers are found) the results of percussion and palpation tests can be of equal or greater value in locating the offending tooth.

Most assaults on the pulp arise from bacterial invasion of dentin. (i.e., caries) As caries progress through the dentin noxious irritants destroy the odontoblastic processes and ultimately penetrate the pulp tissue, lysing cells. This cell death results in the concomitant release of several inflammatory mediators including PgE_2 [38].

Another significant reaction is an increase of white blood cells (WBCs) and extravascular fluids into the confines of the pulp chamber. Two neuropeptides, substance P (sP) and calcitonin gene-related peptide (CGRP) are released and play a major role in altering the perception of pain. These neuropeptides are also reported to be responsible for a lowering of the pain threshold of the afferent nerve fibers resulting in a "hyperalgesia" [39]. When present, they cause edema within the pulp tissues by dilating and increasing the permeability of blood vessels [40].

Neuropeptides are just one group of endogenous chemical mediators released in response to cell lysis. Other mediators include fibrinolytic peptides, kinins, complement fragments, vasoactive amines, lysosomal enzymes, arachidonic acid metabolites, cytokines, and a host of other mediators of immunologic reactions. Some of these mediators are also responsible for lysing pulp cells and once triggered, the level of mediators (that lower the pain threshold) increases to the point that *pain becomes spontaneous*. Once spontaneous aching pain (involvement of C-fibers) occurs stopping or reversing the inflammatory process becomes unlikely and thus the diagnosis "*Irreversible Pulpitis.*"

Prostaglandin E_2 (PgE_2) is produced by the action of cyclooxygenase on arachidonic acid (a product of disrupted cell membranes) and has been shown to lower the pain threshold of afferent fibers in the coronal portion of the pulp. Studies report high concentrations of PgE_2 found in pulps is a marker for "*Irreversible Pulpitis*" [41, 42]. *Concentrating on just this key mediator (PgE_2) provides a simplified paradigm to follow the progression of pulp pain.*

Recall inflammation is the body's expected reaction to a noxious attack. It is prompted by the release of mediators intended to eradicate bacteria and/or dilute toxins. In either case the body responds by sending defense cells, white blood cells (WBCs), and cellular fluids (edema) into the pulp chamber and canal.

Both contribute to an increase of fluid and inflammatory cells within the pulp chamber. The increase in fluid volume results in increased pressure within the chamber that can reasonably account for the continuous aching and throbbing (pulsing) pain typical of irreversible pulpitis. Once "spontaneous or unprovoked pulpal pain" occurs the pulp is presumed to be incapable of healing and deemed "irreversible" [43]. This increase in inflammatory mediators cause a "hyperalgesia" of the C-fibers within the central and radicular pulp tissues. Patients usually respond with prolonged aching pain to thermal challenges and often report being unable to lay flat to sleep or are wakened by an unprovoked throbbing or "pulsing" pain.

The pulse pressure wave generated by the flow of blood through pulp blood vessels has long been proposed as the stimulus for the throbbing pain that arises from the inflamed pulp. However, recent research has challenged this postulate by determining *the rate of the throb differs from the heart rate*. The research showed distinct fractal properties for the tooth and heart. (i.e., throb rate was 44 bpm ± 3 SEM vs. heart rate 72 bpm ± 2 SEM[3] [44].

It is well known that the position of the head in relation to the heart will moderate the pain. (Head above the heart is less painful than head below the heart). This maxim implies a connection between throbbing pain and the pulse pressure wave. As a side note, for over 2000 years the throbbing associated with a toothache was attributed to the pulse wave generated by the heartbeat. More studies are needed in this area to explain this discrepancy in rates.

Another finding suggesting that the throbbing is related to the edema within the pulp is that (in some instances) cold may provide temporary relief. It is common knowledge that the application of cold to an inflamed area can provide relief by reducing swelling (edema) in the area. (Hence the bag of frozen peas in the freezer.)

Cold water or ice may also reduce toothache pain arising from a "partially necrotic pulp" by decreasing pressure if air trapped within the pulp chamber. (See discussion of Aerodontalgia that follows.) This conundrum may account for some of the perplexing thermal test results.

Obtaining satisfactory local anesthesia may be difficult due to edema. If adequate anesthesia cannot be achieved, the patient should be placed on an appropriate antibiotic and appointed to return in 2–3 days. In the meantime, *they should be directed not to place a warm compress to the external area*. Frequent intraoral rinses with warm saline are appropriate. Patients must be instructed to contact the provider or go to the ED if swelling does not improve or function is impaired, especially swallowing or breathing.

Necrobiosis

"Partial pulp necrosis" also referred to as "Necrobiosis" is defined as a condition where some of the pulp has necrosed while a portion of the pulp, further apical in the canal, is still viable but inflamed (i.e., presumably irreversible pulpitis). Pulps undergoing necrobiosis may be difficult to assess because some cases present inconsistent responses to EPTs and/or cold tests [45]. Since the pulp tissue is in the process of dying and retreating from the pulp chamber, it is possible that thermal tests fail to provide a sufficient change in temperature to excite the remaining viable tissue deep in the canal and the EPT may fail due to a void left by the necrotic pulp "preventing continuity" in the high current circuit. (See Chap. 4 Discussion on "current density.")

Patients often report using an OTC toothache remedy or analgesic to relieve their pain. Unfortunately, the use of these products can alter test findings and lead to misdiagnosis based on corrupt information. The fact that a patient sought relief from spontaneous, long duration pulpal pain is sufficient reason to suspect the pulp is irreversibly inflamed and incapable of self-repair. A problem often caused by using OTC remedies is that Diagnostic testing may be invalidated. Endodontic treatment should be considered if the tooth is restorable and contributes to the overall treatment plan.

---

[3] Standard error of the mean.

Aerodontalgia

A necrotic pulp chamber should not react to thermal challenge except in a rare condition known as "Tooth Squeeze." It was first recognized during World War 1 by pilots experiencing tooth pain upon changes in atmospheric pressure as they flew. It was subsequently reported by divers upon rising from the depths. Today it is known as "Barodontalgia" or "Aerodontalgia." Invariably, the condition comes on suddenly from previously asymptomatic teeth.

A patient experiencing aerodontalgia may present in your waiting room and not necessarily at "altitude" as described in Ingle's text. In order to appreciate the physics and physiology contributing to the patients' pain, one needs only to consider Charles "Ideal Gas Laws" linking volume and pressure to absolute temperature. Consider the patient presenting with a cup of ice water and using it to quell his pain. Shortly after taking a sip of the cold water and holding it on the tooth symptoms seem to subside only to return a couple of minutes later.

We are witnessing the cold water cooling air molecules within the confines of the hollow pulp chamber, decreasing their kinetic energy thereby decreasing the pressure exerted on the chamber walls and remaining vital radicular pulp tissue. As the pressure diminishes and pain subsides more air molecules diffuse from the remaining pulp into the void left by necrosed coronal pulp to equalize pressure. As the molecules warm-up kinetic energy increases, exerting pressure on the remaining radicular pulp tissue and the pain returns.

This is a unique condition that is rarely long lasting; rather, it occurs during a transitional period in which the coronal pulp necroses leaving a void, but viable radicular pulp tissue is still intact blocking the apical foramen. For pain to occur the coronal and apical portion of the pulp canal must be sealed to prevent air escaping through an open pulp chamber equalizing pressure. This is not likely to happen if the entire pulp has necrosed allowing loss of pressure through an open apex.

Aerodontalgia may be suspected from a failed pulp cap where the coronal pulp tissues necrose over time and a portion of the radicular pulp remains viable but occludes the apex. It can also occur immediately following restoration of a tooth if there is a void in the pulp chamber and viable tissue at the apex. Use of an OTC temporary stopping restoration may seal a hollow chamber and create an ideal condition for aerodontalgia. However, a temporary stopping may also seal the only way for pus/exudate to escape from a chronic apical abscess (CAA) draining through the open pulp canal. The once painless tooth may suddenly become painful and an acute apical abscess results. Historically, this abscess was labeled a "Phoenix Abscess."

My first experience with Aerodontalgia is worth recounting in the hopes of sparing the reader an embarrassment that has tormented me since it occurred.

Shortly after having been assigned to the Urgent Care Clinic at UFCD, a 22-years-old female presented with periodic severe aching pain from the UR quadrant that had been increasing in intensity over the last couple of days.

Medical history and vitals were non-contributory and within normal limits. The patient denied any parafunctional habits, allergies, or sinus problems. Overall, her dentition had been recently restored and the gingiva was pink and healthy with minimal pocketing and no "food traps."

The only crown was recently placed (2 months ago) on the right maxillary first molar and appeared to be in excellent condition. Panoramic view w/bitewing revealed excellent restorations and no evidence of periapical lucency.

Her **chief complaint** was intense aching/throbbing pain associated with the right side of her face that was brought on when having soup or hot tea. Chewing was not reported to be a problem.

I then started my set routine examining the patient.

External exam was non-contributory, sinuses were not tender to palpation, and there was one palpable (R) submandibular lymph node 3/4 cm Dia. non-tender. TMJ assessment was within normal limits.

Intraoral exam posterior tongue presence of lingual tonsils (WNL), floor of mouth supple, and not tender. vestibular areas all (WNL). Mucosal and gingival tissues all appeared within normal limits. No discomfort reported.

Moving on to the dentition: Despite the patient failing to complain of chewing, I proceeded to tap each cusp on the right side, upper, and lower to rule out a fractured tooth. Percussion was normal for all teeth.

Next was thermal, although the patient complained about heat causing the pain I resorted to the standard "Cold Test" since molding compound was not available in the urgent care clinic. After failing to provoke pain from any tooth in the arch, I turned to the "view box" to study the panoramic image, praying for an epiphany. (Digital imagery was not available at the time.) After what seemed to be an eternity, without any inkling as to the cause of her chief complaint, I turned back to the patient only to see the young lady holding the side of her red face with both hands, in obvious pain, with a tear rolling down from her right eye. Then it happened! The moment I will take to my grave… I asked, sounding with disbelief… "Are you in pain now?"

As the words sprung from my mouth, my self-esteem withered. Not only was I at a loss to diagnose her problem after more than 13 years of private practice experience, but I had followed through with an inquiry that eliminated any question as to my qualifications.

But for every YING there is a YANG, and this situation was not the exception.

YES, my ego was deflated, and it took me back to when I was a child… Question! … As a child did your parents ever put a blown-up balloon in the freezer and show you how it shrank? Then take it out and watch it expand? Mine did!

Well, that was my saving grace! I asked the patient to tell me about the crown and she proceeded to tell me that originally when the dentist filled the tooth, he told her she may need a root canal, but he was going to "treat the nerve" and if she did not have pain in a couple of months he would "have to crown it since the filling was so large." After a couple of months, she was pain free and 2 months ago he placed the crown. It was fine till a few days ago she started to have pain whenever eating something hot. The pain would go away a little while after eating but return periodically each time getting worse. Reporting "Till now, it is so bad I need to have something done."

AND THERE IT WAS…The void left by the necrosing pulp was: "The balloon in the pulp chamber." Expanding when warmed and shrinking when cooled. The difference being that the elastic balloon could expand or contract with the changes in pressure while the pulp canal being ridged cannot adapt to equalize pressure. Therefore, the pressure within the void area of the chamber increased pressing against the remaining vital tissue within the pulp canal.

This is a condition most all of us have witnessed. Recall the patient in your waiting room periodically sipping a cool drink?

Interestingly, the temporary relief is usually followed with an even worse pain minutes after sipping the drink. As the hollow chamber cooled, air molecules entered equalizing the air pressure in the void. As the tooth warmed up the air molecules gained kinetic energy and began to move faster increasing the pressure against the vital tissue remaining in the depth of the pulp canal, provoking an aching throbbing pain by triggering the sensory nerve fibers (C-fibers).

The next time a patient comes into your office sipping a cold drink it may not be caused by a craving for sugar but rather a cry for help.

1.5.3.4 Periapical Periodontium

The periodontal ligament (PDL) is the supportive part of the dental complex and is mainly innervated with C-fibers. Proprioceptive fibers are also present in the PDL facilitating localization. As inflammatory mediators accumulate at the apex the pain threshold of the afferent sensory fibers in the PDL is lowered to the point that normal forces applied to the PDL result in discomfort, i.e., the tooth becomes sensitive to biting forces and percussion.

According to Owatz inflammatory mediators arising from an inflamed pulp initially seep through the apex and initiate a mechanical allodynia of the apical PDL, thereby directing the patient's attention to the offending tooth each time an occlusal force is applied [38]. *A slight difference in response to percussion may be sufficient to identify the offending tooth.* As an infection spreads through the apex, the level of inflammatory mediators (especially PgE_2) increases within the PDL, and the region will become sensitive to palpation.

Initially the inflammatory response includes accumulation of extracellular fluids at the apex, leaving the tooth sensitive to biting and percussion forces. As more fluid (exudate) accumulates at the apex percussion may yield a "thud" sound rather than the characteristic crisp sound normally heard. This accumulation of fluid (edema) is an indication that the periodontitis is progressing on to an abscess. The surrounding tissues will become sensitive to palpation and the tooth depressible in the socket. Any tooth depressible in the socket (Class 3 Mobility) is highly suggestive of an acute apical abscess (AAA).

As the abscess forms the levels of PgE_2 and inflammatory mediators soar in the general area resulting in a diffuse hyperalgesia radiating to the surrounding tissue and cortical bone causing the adjacent area to be painful to palpation as well as percussion [6]. This increase in PgE_2 provokes the continuous aching pain characteristic of C-fiber involvement.

Once there is radiographic evidence of a widened PDL, and the surrounding tissues (especially the cortical bone and periosteum) become sensitive to palpation, (w/o swelling) there is ample reason to assume sufficient cells have lysed resulting in an accumulation of pus at the site and it should be called what it is… an "*abscess*." Once the pus begins to break through the periosteum, a fluctuant swelling will be noted. Prior to breaking through the periosteum, edema (a painful diffuse, firm, swelling in the surrounding soft tissues) is likely to develop. This also is a sign that an abscess is forming but has yet to coalesce to a well-defined area.

An apical abscess should appear as a radiographic lucency at the apex, but it can take up to 12 days for sufficient bone to be destroyed for an abscess to be visible on a radiographic image. It may take longer to break through the cortical bone and periosteum eventually resulting in vestibular swelling or spread through a fascial space. There is no rational reason to wait until swelling is noted in the surrounding soft tissue to refer to this condition as an abscess and start immediate treatment. An accumulation of pus within the cortical bone and periosteum is an "Abscess" despite an absence of localized swelling.

A fascial space infection (FSI) must be treated promptly and aggressively with antibiotics and elimination of the source of infection. A vestibular space infection (VSI) may end in the formation of a sinus tract allowing pus to drain and the swelling diminish. Though not as life threatening as involvement of a FSI, the swelling should be incised and pus drained (I&D), the source of infection eliminated, and patient treated with an appropriate antibiotic.

Occasionally, an asymptomatic chronic apical abscess (CAA) will flare up (revert to an acute phase). Prior to the new terminology adopted by AAE, this return of a chronic lesion to an acute phase was called a "*Phoenix Abscess*" prior to AAE's modified terminology. Before the onset of acute pain AAE identifies this condition as "Pulp Necrosis/Asymptomatic Apical Periodontitis" or if a sinus tract is present a "Chronic Apical Abscess" (CAA) but does not seem to have an identifying term for an acute exacerbation of a long-standing apical lesion other than to call it an "Acute Apical Abscess."

In fact, there is no histologic difference in the cellular infiltrates between a newly formed abscess or one that has reverted from an asymptomatic lesion. The one essential feature of a Phoenix Abscess is the presence of a large apical lucency lending credence to the prior existence of a long-standing chronic lesion that has reverted to an acute stage.

There are three paths that explain an asymptomatic apical lesion becoming acute. The obvious cause is bacterial invasion through an open pulp chamber. The other is bacteria finding their way to the lesion through the blood stream via a process known as *Anachoresis* [46, 47]. This is more likely to happen when the body's defenses are compromised, and resistance lowered. It is the means by which bacteria are believed to infect joint replacements and heart valves. A third mechanism is that initiating endodontic treatment will alter the type of bacteria (anaerobic to aerobic) in a chronic (non-painful) lesion disrupting the balance established by the body with the bacteria and a flare-up ensues [48]. Consider opening the tooth allows oxygen in, killing anaerobes, and releasing endotoxins that disrupt cells and their membranes ultimately contributing to the formation of PgE_2.

One concept to entertain is that a retained root with a pulp canal open to the oral cavity will behave much like a CAA with the canals acting as the sinus tract. Patients may complain of a fowl taste coming from the tooth periodically as the accumulation of pus/extracellular fluids escape via the open canal.

Saliant Points

The previous discussion can be confusing but there are certain principles that will help clarify.

1. Elicited pain forewarns a potential problem.
2. Spontaneous pain portends cell death and a condition the body will not be able to over-come and the involved tissue will likely necrose.
3. A-∂ fibers are associated mainly with dentin and transmit a short-lasting sharp shooting pain.
4. C-fibers associated with the deeper pulp tissue and periodontium will transmit an aching pain when challenged that is likely to be prolonged.
5. Proprioceptive nerve fibers are not found in the pulp but are present in the periodontium.
6. Partial pulp necrosis may account for confusing test results.
7. Reported existent symptoms should be confirmed with proper testing to rule out possible referred pain.
8. Keep in mind not all toothaches are endodontic in origin.
9. Recognize the importance of using the proper terminology when describing pain.
10. It is more important that we appreciated the process causing the patient's complaint as opposed to labeling it.

1.6 Summary

Putting it together: Your diagnosis should be based on clinical findings and the history of the chief complaint. First, determine the source of the symptoms. Because of specialized nerves, one can often determine if the pain is pulpal or periodontal in origin just from the symptoms reported by the patient. Contributing evidence may be collected via diagnostic testing and radiographic imaging.

Diagnosis of a toothache requires a greater understanding of the bio-physiology of dental pain than simply plugging diagnostic findings into a table. An in-depth understanding of the process resulting in pain is needed not only to derive a diagnosis but to also appreciate the process so that false-positive and false-negative tests can be recognized and considered when attempting a diagnosis.

The diagnosis of a toothache should be based on a thorough anamnesis as well as information derived from timely testing properly conducted and interpreted. The accuracy of a diagnosis is enhanced when the diagnostician can provoke the existent chief complaint by testing.

There are two conditions that affect how pulp tissue responds to challenges. They are the extent of injury to the pulp tissue, and its ability to repair the damage. You should note that the intensity and onset of pain are proportional to the level of PgE_2 produced. Formation of PgE_2 is dependent on destruction of cell membranes. Once the tissue has necrosed, and viable cells are no longer available, the level of PgE_2 decreases along with the intensity of pain.

To repeat my original postulate in terms of diagnosis of toothaches, "… Follow the PgE_2."

References

1. Devaraj C, Eswar P. Reasons for use and non-use of dental services among people visiting a dental college hospital in India: a descriptive cross-sectional study. Eur J Dent. 2012;6(4):422–7. PMID: 23077423; PMCID: PMC3474558.
2. Lundy T, Stanley HR. Correlation of pulpal histopathology and clinical symptoms in human teeth subjected to experimental irritation. Oral Surg Oral Med Oral Pathol. 1969;27(2):187–201. https://doi.org/10.1016/0030-4220(69)90172-8. PMID: 5249516.
3. Seltzer S, Rainey E, Gluskin AH. Correlation of scanning electron microscope and light microscope findings in uninflamed and pathologically involved human pulps. Oral Med Oral Pathol. 1977;43(6):910–28. https://doi.org/10.1016/0030-4220(77)90085-8. PMID: 266684.
4. Glickman GN. AAE Consensus conference on diagnostic terminology: background and perspectives. J Endod. 2009;35(12):1619–20. https://doi.org/10.1016/j.joen.2009.09.029. PMID: 19932336.
5. Hargreaves KM, Roszkowski MT, Jackson DL. Pharmacology of peripheral neuropeptides and inflammatory mediator release. Oral Surg Oral Med Oral Pathol. 1994;78(4):503–10. https://doi.org/10.1016/0030-4220(94)90045-0.
6. McNicholas S, Torabinejad M, Blankenship J, Bakland L. The concentration of prostaglandin E2 in human periradicular lesions. J Endod. 1991;17(3):97–100. https://doi.org/10.1016/S0099-2399(06)81737-1.
7. Lin LM, Ricucci D, Saoud TM, Sigurdsson A, Kahler B. Vital pulp therapy of mature permanent teeth with irreversible pulpitis from the perspective of pulp biology. Aust Endod J. 2020;46(1):154–66. https://doi.org/10.1111/aej.12392. Epub 2019 Dec 21.
8. Okeson JP. Non-odontogenic toothache. Northwest Dent. 2000;79(5):37–44.
9. West NX, Lussi A, Seong J, Hellwig E. Dentin hypersensitivity: pain mechanisms and aetiology of exposed cervical dentin. Clin Oral Investig. 2013;17(Suppl 1):S9–19. https://doi.org/10.1007/s00784-012-0887-x. Epub 2012 Dec 9. PMID: 23224116.
10. Jacobsen PL, Bruce G. Clinical dentin hypersensitivity: understanding the causes and prescribing a treatment. J Contemp Dent Pract. 2001;2(1):1–12.
11. Jain N, Gupta A. An insight into neurophysiology of pulpal pain: facts and hypotheses. Korean J Pain. 2013;26(4):347–55. https://doi.org/10.3344/kjp.2013.26.4.347. Epub 2013 Oct 2. PMID: 24156000; PMCID: PMC3800706.
12. Dimitriu B, Vârlan C, Suciu I, Vârlan V, Bodnar D. Current considerations concerning endodontically treated teeth: alteration of hard dental tissues and biomechanical properties following endodontic therapy. J Med Life. 2009;2(1):60–5. PMID: 20108492; PMCID: PMC5051483.
13. Galler KM, Weber M, Korkmaz Y, Widbiller M, Feuerer M. Inflammatory response mechanisms of the dentine-pulp complex and the periapical tissues. Int J Mol Sci. 2021;22(3):1480. https://doi.org/10.3390/ijms22031480. PMID: 33540711; PMCID: PMC7867227.
14. Pashley DH. Dynamics of the pulpo-dentin complex. Crit Rev Oral Biol Med. 1996;7(2):104–33. https://doi.org/10.1177/10454411960070020101. PMID: 8875027.
15. Bender IB. Pulpal pain diagnosis–a review. J Endod. 2000;26(3):175–9. https://doi.org/10.1097/00004770-200003000-00012. PMID: 11199715.
16. Melzack R, Torgerson WS. On the language of pain. Anesthesiology. 1971;34(1):50–9. https://doi.org/10.1097/00000542-197101000-00017.
17. Ferraro EF. Differential diagnosis of orofacial pain. Compend Contin Educ Dent. 1982;3(6):435–9.

18. Melzack R. The McGill Pain Questionnaire: major properties and scoring methods. Pain. 1975;1(3):277–99. https://doi.org/10.1016/0304-3959(75)90044-5. PMID: 1235985.
19. Ricucci D, Loghin S, Siqueira JF. Correlation between clinical and histologic pulp diagnoses. J Endod. 2014;40(12):1932–9. https://doi.org/10.1016/j.joen.2014.08.010. Epub 2014 Oct 12.
20. Thomas K, Robinson H. Oral and dental diagnosis. 5th ed. Philadelphia: W.B. Saunders Company; 1963.
21. Caldeira CL, Barletta FB, Ilha MC, Abrão CV, Gavini G. Pulse oximetry: a useful test for evaluating pulp vitality in traumatized teeth. Dent Traumatol. 2016;32(5):385–9. https://doi.org/10.1111/edt.12279. Epub 2016 May 3.
22. Oskui IZ, Ashtiani MN, Hashemi A, Jafarzadeh H. Effect of thermal stresses on the mechanism of tooth pain. J Endod. 2014;40(11):1835–9. https://doi.org/10.1016/j.joen.2014.06.014. Epub 2014 Aug 27.
23. Murray GM. Referred pain, allodynia and hyperalgesia. J Am Dent Assoc. 2009;140(9):1122–4. https://doi.org/10.14219/jada.archive.2009.0339.
24. Sandkühler J. Models and mechanisms of hyperalgesia and allodynia. Physiol Rev. 2009;89(2):707–58. https://doi.org/10.1152/physrev.00025.2008.
25. Seale NS, McIntosh JE, Taylor AN. Pulpal reaction to bleaching of teeth in dogs. J Dent Res. 1981;60(5):948–53. https://doi.org/10.1177/00220345810600051701. PMID: 6938571.
26. Morgan J. Dentin hypersensitivity from bleaching. Inside Dent. 2014;10:4.
27. Jorgensen MG, Carroll WB. Incidence of tooth sensitivity after home whitening treatment. J Am Dent Assoc. 2002;133(8):1076–82. https://doi.org/10.14219/jada.archive.2002.0332.
28. Lavigne SE, Gutenkunst LS, Williams KB. Effects of tartar-control dentifrice on tooth sensitivity: a pilot study. J Dent Hyg. 1997;71(3):105–11.
29. https://en.wikipedia.org/wiki/Allodynia.
30. Mrinalini, Sodvadiya UB, Hegde MN, et al. An update on dentinal hypersensitivity aetiology to management – a review. J Evol Med Dent Sci. 2021;10(37):3289–93. https://doi.org/10.14260/jemds/2021/667.
31. Brännström M. The hydrodynamic theory of dentinal pain: sensation in preparations, caries and dentinal crack syndrome. J Endod. 1986;12:453–7. https://doi.org/10.1016/S0099-2399(86)80198-4.
32. Miglani S, Aggarwal V, Ahuja B. Dentin hypersensitivity: recent trends in management. J Conserv Dent. 2010;13(4):218–24. https://doi.org/10.4103/0972-0707.73385. PMID: 21217949; PMCID: PMC3010026.
33. Hargreaves KM, Cohen S. Cohen's pathways of the pulp. 10th ed. St. Louis: Mosby; 2010. p. 510.
34. Huang GT, Gronthos S, Shi S. Mesenchymal stem cells derived from dental tissues vs. those from other sources: their biology and role in regenerative medicine. J Dent Res. 2009;88(9):792–806. https://doi.org/10.1177/0022034509340867. PMID: 19767575; PMCID: PMC2830488.
35. https://en.wikipedia.org/wiki/Pulp_(tooth).
36. Närhi M, Jyväsjärvi E, Virtanen A, Huopaniemi T, Ngassapa D, Hirvonen T. Role of intradental A- and C-type nerve fibres in dental pain mechanisms. Proc Finn Dent Soc. 1992;88(1):507–16.
37. Batista PJ, Pantera EA. Principles of endodontic diagnosis. Decis Dent. 2020;6(4):9–10.
38. Owatz CB, Khan AA, Schindler WG, Schwartz SA, Keiser K, Hargreaves KM. The incidence of mechanical allodynia in patients with irreversible pulpitis. J Endod. 2007;33(5):552–6. https://doi.org/10.1016/j.joen.2007.01.023. Epub 2007 Mar 6.
39. Ma W. Chronic prostaglandin E2 treatment induces the synthesis of the pain-related peptide substance P and calcitonin gene-related peptide in cultured sensory ganglion explants. J Neurochem. 2010;115(2):363–72. https://doi.org/10.1111/j.1471-4159.2010.06927.x. Epub 2010 Aug 25.
40. Abd-Elmeguid A, Yu DC. Dental pulp neurophysiology: part 1. Clinical and diagnostic implications. J Can Dent Assoc. 2009;75(1):55–9.

41. Torabinejad M, Bakland LK. Prostaglandins: their possible role in the pathogenesis of pulpal and periapical diseases, part 2. J Endod. 1980;6(10):769–76. https://doi.org/10.1016/S0099-2399(80)80107-5.
42. Cohen JS, Reader A, Fertel R, Beck M, Meyers WJ. A radioimmunoassay determination of the concentrations of prostaglandins E2 and F2alpha in painful and asymptomatic human dental pulps. J Endod. 1985;11(8):330–5. https://doi.org/10.1016/s0099-2399(85)80039-x. PMID: 3863874.
43. Petrini M, Ferrante M, Ciavarelli L, Brunetti L, Vacca M, Spoto G. Prostaglandin E2 to diagnose between reversible and irreversible pulpitis. Int J Immunopathol Pharmacol. 2012;25(1):157–63. https://doi.org/10.1177/039463201202500118. PMID: 22507328.
44. Mirza AF, Mo J, Holt JL, Kairalla JA, Heft MW, Ding M, Ahn AH. Is there a relationship between throbbing pain and arterial pulsations? J Neurosci. 2012;32(22):7572–6. https://doi.org/10.1523/JNEUROSCI.0193-12.2012. PMID: 22649235; PMCID: PMC3376713.
45. Jafarzadeh H, Abbott PV. Review of pulp sensibility tests. Part I: general information and thermal tests. Int Endod J. 2010;43(9):738–62. https://doi.org/10.1111/j.1365-2591.2010.01754.x. Epub 2010 Jul 1.
46. Dezan E, Holland R, Consolaro A, Ciesielski FIN, Jardim EG. Experimentally induced anachoresis in the periapical region after root canal filling. Int J Odontostomatol. 2012;6(1):5–10.
47. Robinson HG, Boling LR. The anachoretic effect in pulpitis. I bacteriologic studies. J Dent Assoc. 1941;28(1):268–82.
48. Carrotte P. Endodontics: part 3. Treatment of endodontic emergencies. Br Dent J. 2004;197(6):299–305. https://doi.org/10.1038/sj.bdj.4811641.

Progression of Pulp Disease 2

2.1 Introduction

Over the years, there have been attempts to adopt a universal nomenclature for pulp pathosis based on histologic findings to clinical symptoms. Unfortunately, the histologic approach did little to explain the cause of the problem prior to extraction and microscopic examination of the remaining contents of the pulp. Grossman's "Classification of Pulp Disease" reflected the end product of the disease at the time of diagnosis and treatment. There is little attention to the biophysiology of pain.

Current terminology adopted by the American Association of Endodontists (AAE) also identifies "snapshots" of static odontogenic conditions based on existent symptoms but also does little to explain the progression of pulp disease. The stated purpose for this latest classification is to facilitate communication between referring dentists and endodontists and direct proper treatment by deriving a diagnosis based on existent clinical tests and symptoms. Conspicuously missing is the progression of changes in pain as the pulp undergoes its demise. An understanding of this progression facilitates diagnosis. It is important to appreciate odontogenic pain is not a static condition, rather an ever-changing process that is affected by a number of independent conditions including OTC analgesics and palliatives that can alter test results, i.e., the use of eugenol or benzocaine can obtund pain originating from an inflamed pulp, i.e., diminish the response to a diagnostic test. Failure to consider a history of spontaneous pain and/or use of analgesics or topical remedies could lead to a flawed diagnosis.

This work conveys an abridged bio-physical exploration of the process that accounts for the major factors triggering symptoms a patient may experience from a diseased pulp. It is not meant to challenge the present diagnostic paradigm as proposed by AAE, rather to help dentists understand the etiology of and temporal changes in symptoms associated with a dying pulp.

E. Lado, R. Caudle, *Pathway to Diagnosis and Management of Toothaches*,
https://doi.org/10.1007/978-3-031-75262-9_2

2.1.1 Normal Pulp (Refer to Fig. 2.1)

It is important to note dentinal sensitivity (DS) and dental hypersensitivity (DH) are characteristics of pain attributed to dentin and is not necessarily interconnected to an inflammation of the pulp. Dentinal pain is often attendant to stimulation of specific sensory fibers (a-∂ nerve fibers) and not to lysis of cell membranes and formation of prostaglandin E_2 (PgE_2) with one possible exception (*Dental Hypersensitivity*) to be discussed.

The dental pulp is the innermost part of the tooth that accommodates nerves and blood supply. It is protected by enamel and dentin that when decayed or damaged can result in exposure of the pulp. An exposed pulp is susceptible to infection and necrosis that accounts for most "toothaches." Prompt treatment is often needed to alleviate the patient's discomfort and risk of advancing infection.

The pulp is innervated mainly by two major types of sensory nerves (a-∂ and C-fibers). A-∂ fibers transmit sharp shooting pain while C-fibers transmit a longer aching pain. The a-∂ fibers are concentrated in the coronal portion of the pulp and extend into the dentinal tubules. On the other hand, C-fibers are found deeper in the pulp canal. Thus, in healthy pulps a-∂ fibers are the first nerves to respond to an external challenge with sharp pain.

Odontoblastic processes occupy dental tubules and when stimulated odontoblasts form tertiary and/or reparative dentin. If odontoblast processes in dental tubules are overwhelmed by irritants, they lyse leaving a hollow tubule through which irritants can easily penetrate to the pulp. (In effect, they become micro-exposures.) When the odontoblast membranes are destroyed, arachidonic acid (a

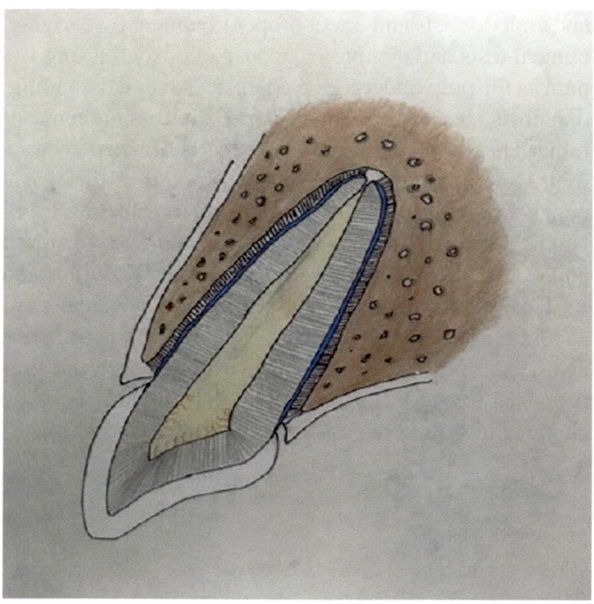

Fig. 2.1 Normal pulp*.
*Old terminology

precursor of Prostaglandins including PgE_2) is released. PgE_2 is known to lower the pain threshold of sensory nerves. Initially, PgE_2 lowers the pain threshold of the a-∂ fibers responsible for a sharp "shooting" pain. As the pain mediator spreads toward the apex, the pain threshold of the C-fibers is lowered, and a prolonged aching pain will prevail. Once the aching pain becomes spontaneous, it is presumed that sufficient cells have been lysed limiting the ability of the pulp to recover (Table 2.1).

2.1.2 Inflamed Pulp

2.1.2.1 Reversible Pulpitis (Refer to Fig. 2.2)

Reversible pulpitis is an inflammatory response of the dental pulp triggered by an insult to pulp tissue [1]. Insults to the tissue include irritants such as acidic foods (i.e., citrus and vinegar), caustic chemicals found in restorative materials, etching agents, chelating agents (found in tarter control dentifrices), tooth whitening agents, toxins produced by bacteria, heat generated during cavity preparation and more (Table 2.2).

Caustic irritants such as bleaching agents have been shown to cause an inflammatory response in pulps of dogs' teeth [2]. There is ample reason to expect this to be the case in human pulps since it is well known that human teeth often become hypersensitive for a period of time following bleaching.

Frictional heat generated during cavity preparation may also destroy odontoblasts preventing formation of protective dentin eventually leaving the pulp incapable of self-repair. It is critical that a coolant is used when preparing a tooth with a high-speed drill.

Parenthetically, repeated stimulation of the a-∂ fibers may result in increased sensitivity (an allodynia, in which pain is caused by a repeated stimulus that does not normally elicit pain and is not characterized by the production of prostaglandins.) Unless preventive measures are taken to eliminate the irritant and protect the open tubules, pain may become so annoying that the patient opts to have root canal treatment or extraction despite the absence of infection.

Irritants can initiate development of tertiary dentin in healthy pulps thereby walling-off the vital pulp tissue for an insult. Failure to do so will often result in

Table 2.1 Response and clinical findings associated with a normal pulp

No spontaneous pulpal pain A sharp response may be elicited by thermal stimulus	Response should be of short duration without a prolonged aching pain Exposed dentin may be sensitive[a]	Expected to respond to EPT unless performed on deciduous or newly erupted teeth with wide open apex. See Chap. 4
Normal response to thermal challenges	No contributory history of dental pain	No abnormal radiographic findings

[a] In accordance with Brännström's theory of pain, exposed dentin can display an exaggerated response to air, thermal, and caustic irritants. Dentin can also become non-responsive if sclerotic/tertiary dentin forms walling-off pulp tissue from external stimuli. But pain from a healthy pulp should be strictly elicited and short duration.

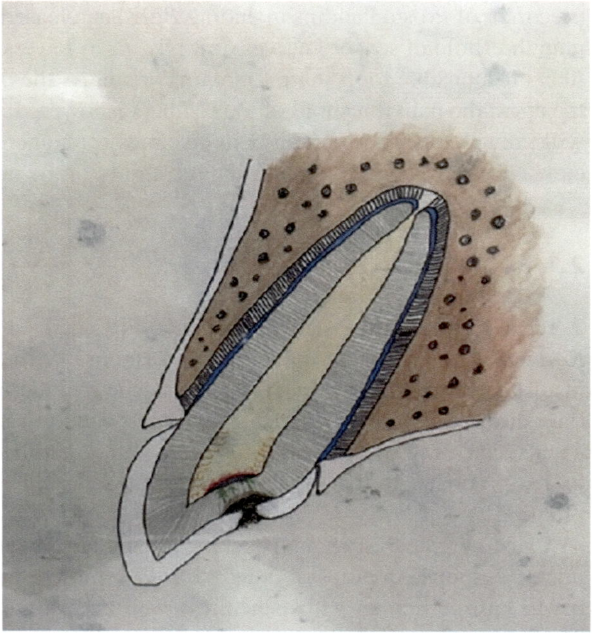

Fig. 2.2 Reversible pulpitis* (Allodynia?). *Old terminology

Table 2.2 Clinical findings associated with reversible pulpitis

No spontaneous pain	Slightly prolonged and exaggerated sharp pain to thermal stimulus	Mainly ∂ fibers are stimulated
Exaggerated response to thermal challenges	Large/caustic restoration, caries, bleaching or whitening agents	Exposed or cracked dentin, caries

reversible pulpitis (RP) (beginning inflammation) progressing on to an irreversible condition if pulp tissue cannot heal and the cause eliminated. Irreversible pulpitis (IP) is characterized by eventual necrosis of the pulp. The IP may be symptomatic (SIP) or asymptomatic (AIP), that advances rapidly or slowly. It is recognized as a progressing "partial pulp necrosis" or "necrobiosis."

Diagnostic testing may be problematic. Unless there is a history of spontaneous pain, one should address the problem conservatively. Suggest the use of desensitizing toothpastes specially targeted at sensitive teeth and avoid all whiteners and tarter control toothpastes. The dentist may recommend restoration or application of a product designed to seal off the open tubules. Spontaneous pulp pain is a strong indication that an irreversible pulpitis has developed rendering the pulp incapable of self-repair with root canal treatment (RTC) or extraction indicated.

When conducting pulp tests, consider the patients' body language not just their verbal response. Diagnostic tests are not infallible, they require skilled execution and interpretation taking all related findings into consideration, i.e., tolerance to pain can vary considerably from person to person as well as from day to day, so the actual reported pain is a subjective finding and deserves some consideration but not the sole criteria on which to base a diagnosis (see Chap. 4).

Since the pulp does not contain proprioceptive nerve fibers, percussion is not an appropriate test to determine status of the "pulp." It is helpful in identifying the suspect tooth if inflammatory mediators (PgE_2) have seeped through the apex lowering of the pain threshold of the sensory C-fibers located in the PDL, resulting in a "Symptomatic Apical Periodontitis (SAP)."

Analgesics are rarely needed to relieve pain caused by allodynia or reversible pulpitis since pain is neither prolonged nor spontaneous. If the patient has resorted to analgesics, consider the likelihood the patient has experienced prolonged, spontaneous pain and that the infection could be spreading past the apical foramen. Failure to respond to thermal testing or electric pulp tester (EPT) is an indication that the pulp has necrosed beyond the range of a reliable test and may result in a false negative leading to a misdiagnosis. Viable tissue may be located deeper in the canal and placing a file without anesthetizing the tooth may result in an unpleasant surprise. The following presents various causes and stages of pulp pathosis.

2.1.2.2 Partial Pulp Necrosis: (Necrobiosis) (Refer to Fig. 2.3)

There are two paths the pulp may follow in the process of dying. One path leads to a painful "*Symptomatic Irreversible Pulpitis*" (*SIP*) while the other becomes a painless condition "*Asymptomatic Irreversible Pulpitis*" (*AIP*). In either case, the pulp eventually necroses leaving the chamber/canal devoid of tissue.

Since most pulps die starting from the coronal portion and move toward the apex, pulp tests and symptoms may yield conflicting results due to a void isolating the

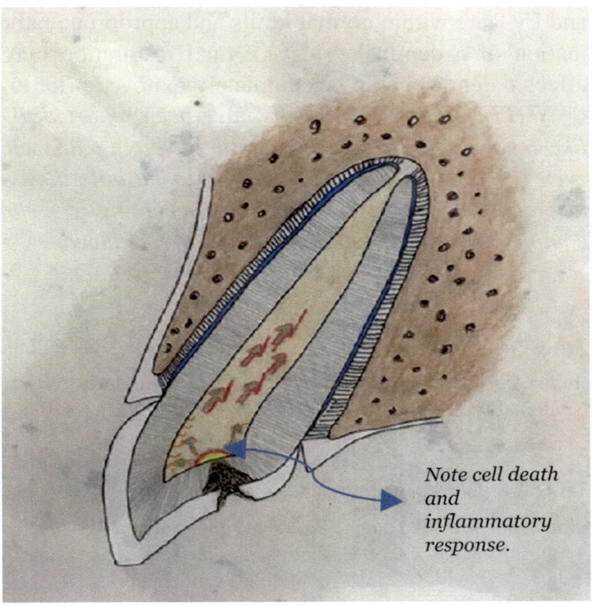

Fig. 2.3 Symptomatic irreversible pulpitis (SIP). Irreversible pulpitis (IP)*. *Old terminology

remaining vital pulp from the test challenge. This process of dying (called *Partial Pulp Necrosis* or *Necrobiosis*) accounts for some of the questionable test results.

As the pulp retreats from the pulp chamber, it becomes more difficult to access the remaining vital pulp with diagnostic tests. Thus, a tooth with vital pulp tissue deep in the canal may test non-reactive yet when instrumentation approaches the working depth patients may experience excruciating pain. One may conclude that part of the pulp remaining in the canal is vital.

An accurate diagnosis is contingent upon putting all the pieces of the puzzle together and not reliance on ad hoc symptoms and arbitrary diagnostic tests and interpretations.

"Symptomatic Irreversible Pulpitis" (SIP) (Refer to Fig. 2.3)

Symptomatic Irreversible Pulpitis (SIP) is a sign that pulp tissue is dying, and the level of PgE_2 increases greatly resulting in spontaneous pulpal pain. Root canal treatment (RCT) must be considered if the tooth is to be retained. A history of spontaneous pulpal pain precludes the option to pulp cap except for recently erupted teeth with open apices since these teeth have a better potential for survival by forming a dentinal bridge that will protect the pulp. A caveat is that the necrotic tissue must be removed, and the capping agent placed directly on healthy pulp tissue for new dentin to form. This is best suited for a fresh mechanical exposure with a prior history excluding spontaneous pain (Tables 2.3 and 2.4).

It has been noted that viable healthy pulp tissue must be in direct contact with a pulp capping agent for new dentin to form [3]. Indirect pulp caps may be performed on reversible pulpitis to allow apposition of a thicker wall of dentin so as to prevent exposure of the pulp when remaining caries is removed and a final restoration placed [4]. Once the tooth has remained asymptomatic for 3-4 months, diagnostic testing and EPT are within normal limits and appropriate radiographic imaging shows formation of a dentinal bridge, a final restoration may be placed. The remaining affected dentin should be completely removed prior to placing the final restoration.

NOTE: *Mesenchymal cells have been reported to transform into odontoblast-like cells capable of forming dentin in young pulps with an ample blood supply. So even if the odontoblasts are destroyed initially these transformed cells may form new dentin* [5]. *The chance of this occurring is greatly reduced once the apex is completely formed, and the blood supply reduced.*

Table 2.3 Common causes of Symptomatic Irreversible Pulpitis

Injury (mechanical exposure, frictional/chemical burn)	Bacterial intrusion (pathologic necrosis)	Loss of blood supply (trauma)

Table 2.4 Clinical findings associated with a SIP

Spontaneous aching pain requiring analgesics for relief	Prolonged and exaggerated sharp pain to thermal that progresses on to unprovoked continuous aching pain	a-∂ fibers are initially stimulated followed by C-fibers

NOTE: *A large restoration/caries may interfere with diagnostic testing by insulating the pulp from the challenge. Also, it is important to consider the anodyne effects of a sedative restoration such as zinc oxide and eugenol when interpreting pulp test findings.*

Common Causes of Symptomatic Irreversible Pulpitis

1. *Mechanical exposure*: of a pulp during cavity preparation can lead to an uncomfortable discussion with the patient. The decision to pulp cap, extract, or provide endodontic treatment should be discussed prior to starting treatment and preparations made in advance to avoid last minute discussions. Several factors must be considered besides cost such as restorability, long term prognosis, and compatibility with the overall treatment plan.

   One must appreciate that for a direct pulp cap to succeed the pulp must be healthy and the capping agent (i.e., calcium hydroxide) must be placed in direct contact with viable pulp tissue. If the tooth exhibited symptoms of an irreversible pulpitis, the direct or indirect pulp cap should not be attempted unless infected tissue can be removed, and the capping agent is placed directly on healthy pulp tissue. This procedure is best offered to young patients with recently erupted teeth and open apex. It usually entails the removal of the affected coronal pulp, leaving viable tissue in the canals and capping the healthy tissue with a calcium hydroxide capping agent. The pulp in the canal should appear pink without hemorrhage. A bleeding pulp is likely to be inflamed and therefore a poor candidate for a pulp cap.

   Following pulp capping, a tooth may mimic symptoms of reversible pulpitis and then die quietly (without further symptoms). A permanent restoration with complete removal of the caries may be considered if all subsequent tests are found to be within normal limits and the history does not include spontaneous or prolonged pain requiring analgesics or OTC remedies. Prior to placing the final restoration, radiographic imaging and vitality tests should be performed after 120 days to evaluate and confirm a dentinal bridge has formed and the pulp is still healthy.

   An "indirect pulp cap" is often attempted to avoid exposure and allow time for reparative dentin to be laid down. Again, the tooth must not have exhibited irreversible symptoms for a pulp capping procedure to work.

   An indirect pulp cap should be considered a temporary measure allowing time for the odontoblasts to deposit additional reparative dentin to protect the pulp from exposure upon removal of the remaining caries and placement of the final restoration. Leaving the capping material as a base violates the cavity preparation procedure that calls for removal of all infected dentin. There has been some belief that sealing caries under the restoration prevents bacterial growth by cutting off the supply of nutrients for the bacteria. This is a flawed supposition in that bacteria will get their required nutrients from interstitial fluid taken up through the dental tubules if they have not been sealed by reparative dentin.

   Quite often I have heard recurrent caries under a restoration blamed on a leaky margin. I find it amazing how the bacteria worked their way down the side of the restoration without causing caries but waited till they got under the restoration to begin their damage. Occam's razor, a principle attributed to fourteenth century friar William of Ockham says… that if you have two competing ideas to explain the same phenomenon, you should prefer the simpler one. I put my money on "remaining infected caries."

2. *Frictional or caustic-chemical burn*: will progressively necrose pulp tissue if not prevented or eliminated. Frictional burn is likely to occur from inadequate cooling of the bur during cavity preparation. Chemical burns may be caused by improper curing of polymer restorative materials or acids used to etch a preparation for a polymer restoration. Improperly cured restorations may leach caustic chemicals into dentinal tubules causing cell lysis. As pulp cells progressively necrose, PgE_2 production lowers the pain threshold of the a-∂ and C-fibers resulting in spontaneous, exaggerated, and prolonged pain progressively necrosing the pulp tissue.

   The pulp can follow two possible paths in response to a caustic agent. Either the pulp tissue will necrose or the dentin will become denatured and dentinoclasts will phagocytize it as if it were a foreign body. This internal resorption, also known as Pink Tooth of Mummery, appears pink because the thin layer of remaining dentin allows light to be reflected through the enamel.

   The necrosis path may develop slowly and without symptoms or rapidly should it become infected by circulating bacteria. This process of bacteria invading a compromised area is recognized as "Anachoresis" [6, 7]. The process also accounts for bacterial growth in a compromised surgical site such as an artificial joint or an endocarditis resulting from a defective heart valve.

3. *Bacterial invasion*: As bacteria and their toxins penetrate the dentinal tubules, odontoblastic processes are lysed and release arachidonic acid. Reaction of arachidonic acid with cyclooxygenase produces prostaglandin E_2 (PgE_2) that lowers the reactive threshold of sensory nerve fibers. As the amount of PgE_2 increases, the pain threshold of the a-∂ and C-fibers is lowered, and the response to stimulation becomes pronounced and prolonged.

   Once the bacteria reach the pulp a pulpal abscess develops, the odontoblasts are destroyed and are no longer available to produce secondary dentin. At this point, a pulp capping procedure will not succeed on a fully developed tooth. (See previous notes on pulp caps under Symptomatic Irreversible pulpitis.)

   As the pulp necroses and cells continue to be destroyed, PgE_2 concentrations increase and travel deeper into the pulp where C-fibers predominate. C-fibers transmit an aching pain. In time, the level of PgE_2 increases, the pain threshold is reduced, and the aching pain increases in intensity, eventually becoming prolonged and spontaneous.

   Spontaneous pulp pain is one of the more reliable symptoms that indicates the pulp is necrosing. As mentioned, response to thermal and electric testing have limitations. Since the mean arterial pressure within the pulp increases, it is very common for this tooth to hurt more when lying down (see discussion on pulse pressure Chap. 1, p. 5–6, 17–18).

It is common for a patient to complain about thermal changes provoking pain that is not provoked when testing. This occurs as the pulp progressively necroses in the chamber, but vital tissue remains deeper in the pulp canal. This process of pulp degradation (known as partial pulp necrosis or necrobiosis) often confounds interpretation of test results by obstructing transmission of thermal and electric challenges to the remaining pulp.

4. *Trauma*: If the blood supply is severed at the apex, the pulp will die quickly. But if the fracture occurs higher toward the crown, it will undergo a slower death and exhibit symptoms suggestive of an Irreversible pulpitis. Blood may accumulate in the pulp canal and enter the dentinal tubules (See Chap. 3). As the RBCs break down, the dentin is stained and ultimately results in a dark (discolored) tooth. (Not to be confused with "Pink Tooth of Mummery.")

   The void left by necrotic pulp tissue is not capable of transmitting electrical or thermal changes. The pain patients experience from a split root is mainly associated with an inflammation of tissues approximating the apex. The coronal tissue has most likely died and any pain from tests applied to the coronal portion is from the PDL. Intermittent radiographic evaluation of the apical pulp is warranted since the pulp tissue may take some time to completely necrose. Pulp-testing, immediately following trauma, is not reliable since the surrounding tissues are injured and the pain thresholds of the surrounding sensory nerves are greatly reduced due to the presence of inflammatory mediators. Also, the remaining dying tissue or blood in the pulp canal may conduct an electric charge through the apex resulting in a positive reading that could be interpretated that the pulp is "vital."

   Follow-up pulp-testing should be done once surrounding tissues have had a chance to heal and the pulp has had a chance to recover or completely necrose. One week following the incident is a reasonable time to postpone testing unless the patient complains of painful symptoms in the interim.

   Vitality testing is suggested again at 2 weeks and again at 3 months following the incident to confirm the pulp has survived or necrosed. If tests are inconclusive, repeat in 3 more months unless symptoms arise sooner. The health of the pulp and presence of tooth fractures should be checked prior to placing any final restoration such as a crown (refer to Table 3.1 in Chap. 3).

2.1.2.3 Asymptomatic Irreversible Pulpitis (AIP)

1. ***Programed cell death (Apoptosis)***

   Pulp tissue may undergo a slow death due to lysis of cells injured by mechanical, chemical, or traumatic insults w/o contagion by bacteria. This is not uncommon when considering teeth with mechanical exposures or pulps that have been chemically burned with acid used to etch dentinal surfaces prior to placement of "Bonded" restorations. Initially, there will likely be stimulated pain from a-∂ fibers that will fade as the cells die. Patients are likely to complain of sharp pain upon having something cold. This sensitivity dissipates with time. Either the pulp heals or undergoes apoptosis.

As the number of cells that die diminishes, production of PgE_2 also diminishes. In fact, the levels of PgE_2 may be so low that the pain threshold of the neural receptors (C-fibers) is not achieved, and spontaneous pain will be barely perceived if at all. This process is likely to progress till the entire pulp has necrosed. The reason for the slow death of cells is that the initial cause of lysis is no longer present, so the remaining live cells just die off slowly due to a homeostatic imbalance caused by the initial assault on the pulp. This is usually associated with a sterile assault. If pathogens are the cause, it would be unlikely that the pulp will die quietly. In fact, the conditions would be ideal for a bacterial bloom and a dramatic increase in cell death and production of PgE_2 resulting in a symptomatic irreversible pulpitis (SIP)

2. ***Pink tooth of mummery***

   If the pulp fails to protect itself from an irritant, it will continue to undergo changes. Besides the programmed death of cells, here are 2 unique conditions that present as asymptomatic irreversible pulpitis (AIP). First is tooth of mummery, where dentin is denatured and phagocytized by dentinoclasts as if it were a foreign body (internal resorption) and the pulp is replaced with granulation tissue that will eventually necrose. It has been documented that this process may be initiated by a variety of stimuli such as including pulp capping, trauma, extreme heat produced during high-speed preparation, caustic irritants (i.e., acid etching and other irritants) applied to dentin or toxins released by bacteria found in caries. As with apoptosis, unless sufficient cells die rapidly the level of PgE_2 produced may be insufficient to lower the pain threshold significantly for the pulp to exhibit spontaneous pain. The inflammatory response of the pulp reacts to the denatured dentin as if it were a foreign body and begins to eat it away.

   The tooth appears pink because a thin layer of dentin underlying enamel allows light to pass through from a vital, albeit unhealthy pulp. It is well known that internal bleaching can result in external cervical resorption of dentin [8]. It is interesting that resorption occurs in dentin but not enamel. This is most likely due to the inorganic nature of enamel.

3. ***Pulp polyp***

   A pulp polyp, also known as chronic hyperplastic pulpitis, is a reaction of the dental pulp in which granulation tissue overwhelms inflamed pulp tissue in response to a persistent low-grade infection. It is characterized by an overgrowth of granulation tissue outside the boundary of a tooth's pulp chamber. Due to a lack of intra-pulpal pressure in the open lesion pulp, necrosis does not occur quickly as would be expected. A good vascular supply and lack of immune resistance is required for its development. This condition is more commonly seen in molar teeth of children and young adults with wide open apexes and rarely in older patients with restricted apexes. The open apex allows sufficient nutrients to reach the tissue within the pulp to maintain vitality albeit granulation tissue.

   At some point, the pulp polyp "Necroses" as its' blood supply diminishes due to inflammation and/or an abscess forms at the apex.

4. ***Aerodontalgia/Barodontalgia*** (Refer to Chap. 1, p. 19)

It is not uncommon to see a patient in pain sipping on an ice drink while waiting to be examined. Cold tests can present conflicting results when testing an inflamed pulp. It is possible for cold to relieve pain just as a cold compress is used to reduce swelling from a contusion. It is reasonable to assume if there is edema within an abscessed pulp, an application of something cold could provide temporary relief by reducing swelling as with a contusion.

Cold can also provide relief if air is trapped in the pulp chamber as witnessed by a patient periodically sipping cold water to calm a painful tooth. This was first noted during WWI by pilots and later by divers where barometric pressures affected the air pressure in a void within the pulp chamber. It was called "Tooth Squeeze." Today, the term "Aerodontalgia" is used to identify a unique situation where air is trapped in a pulp chamber that is sealed by a restoration with vital pulp tissue remaining in the root occluding egress through the apical foramen.

According to Charles Gas Laws, pressure is proportional to temperature. When air in the pulp chamber is cooled, the pressure within the void diminishes, and the pressure on the remaining pulp tissue at the apex is relieved and thus pain is diminished. In order to maintain an equilibrium in the chamber, more air molecules enter the void. As the tooth warms back up and molecular movement speeds-up, the pressure increases exerting a force against the remaining viable tissue blocking the apex and pain returns. The patient reaches for another sip of ice water to cool it down again, slowing the molecules thereby reducing the pressure against the remaining viable tissues. This is a classic case of aerodontalgia, and it creates a vicious cycle of pain.

Coincidentally, heat can provoke pain by increasing the pressure in a sealed chamber as previously described. This patient will often complain that hot coffee or soup aggravates the pain, conversely relieved when having something cold (i.e., ice cream).

2.1.3 "Necrotic Pulp" (Refer to Fig. 2.4)

Once the pulp completely necroses, all symptoms related to the vital pulp should subside. It is common for multi-rooted teeth to have complete necrosis in one or more canals but still test positive to electric pulp test and thermal challenge if viable tissue remains in one or more of the other canals. This would be considered, as mentioned before, as a "Partial Pulp Necrosis."

An important point to keep in mind is that the hollow pulp chamber remaining after the pulp has necrosed is not biocompatible. The void presents an ideal environment for anaerobic bacteria to thrive. Should anaerobes find their way there, there is no protective cellular response available. The reason it is ideal for anaerobes is that RBCs that carry oxygen do not circulate in the void and defense cells (WBCs) will not aggregate unless the bacteria have overwhelmed the perimeter defense of the void.

Painful symptoms from the tooth complex where the pulp has completely necrosed arise from the PDL and will be discussed in Chap. 5.

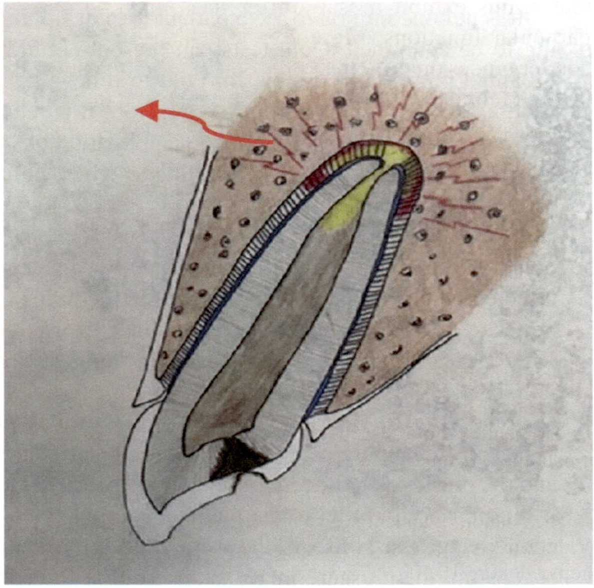

Fig. 2.4 Necrotic pulp/acute apical abscess NP/AAA*. *Old terminology

1. *Sterile Necrosis*
2. *Luxated/Avulsed Tooth*
3. *Caustic Irritant*

Salient Points

- Pulps may die without bacterial invasion from the following causes: *sterile necrosis, luxated or avulsed tooth, caustic irritant, acid etch, frictional heat.*
- When diagnosing a toothache, it is important to consider all available information pertinent to the chief complaint, ensuring the findings are coherent with the condition, e.g., identifying a tooth treated with endo as the offending tooth while the chief complaint includes sensitivity to cold would not be likely to fit the scenario. You must attempt to identify the cause for thermal sensitivity if in fact it pertains to the chief complaint or arises from a proximate tooth.
- Cracked teeth may present a variety of symptoms depending on the type of fracture, the fractures involving the pulp will likely present with irreversible pulpitis or a necrotic pulp while fractures through just the enamel and dentin may only present with a reversible pulpitis. Treatment is highly dependent on the extent of the fracture (refer to Chap. 3).
- Consider the temporal nature of pulp disease. Symptoms change with time, so it is important to establish how the symptoms have changed over time and to attempt to duplicate the existent symptoms with diagnostic challenges.

- Bear in mind dental pulps lack proprioceptive fibers and are likely to refer pain to the opposing arch.... never to the arch on the contralateral side.
- Partial pulp necrosis (necrobiosis) accounts for some of the misleading pulp test results.
- Spontaneous pulpal pain is the most reliable symptom of irreversible pulpitis.
- Thermal testing is valued for its ability to identify the suspect tooth.
- When evaluating the pulp status, you should conduct tests that provoke the chief complaint to ensure the offending tooth is identified.
- Tooth pain may be associated with an inflamed sinus or even referred pain from the heart (angina). When a cause cannot be pinpointed alternative sources of the pain must be investigated.

References

1. Cohen JS, Reader A, Fertel R, Beck M, Meyers WJ. A radioimmunoassay determination of the concentrations of prostaglandins E2 and F2 alpha in painful and asymptomatic human dental pulps. J Endod. 1985;11(8):330–5. https://doi.org/10.1016/s0099-2399(85)80039-x.
2. Seale NS, McIntosh JE, Taylor AN. Pulpal reaction to bleaching of teeth in dogs. J Dent Res. 1981;60(5):948–53. https://doi.org/10.1177/00220345810600051701.
3. Stanley HR. Human pulp response to operative dental procedures. Gainesville: Storter Printing Co. Inc.; 1976. p. 43.
4. Ibid, p. 33.
5. Huang GT, Gronthos S, Shi S. Mesenchymal stem cells derived from dental tissues vs. those from other sources: their biology and role in regenerative medicine. J Dent Res. 2009;88(9):792–806. https://doi.org/10.1177/0022034509340867. PMID: 19767575; PMCID: PMC2830488.
6. Dezan E, Holland R, Consolaro A, Ciesielski FIN, Jardim EG. Experimentally induced anachoresis in the periapical region after root canal filling. Int J Odontostomatol. 2012;6(1):5–10.
7. https://en.wiktionary.org/wiki/anachoresis.
8. Lado EA, Stanley HR, Weisman MI. Cervical resorption in bleached teeth. Oral Surg Oral Med Oral Pathol. 1983;55(1):78–80. https://doi.org/10.1016/0030-4220(83)90310-9.

Cracked Tooth Syndrome

3

3.1 Introduction

Cracked tooth syndrome is one of the more challenging diagnoses you will encounter during your practice of dentistry. Symptoms may not present distinct and consistent patterns, rather they vary pending length of time from initial onset, duration of fracture, the status of the pulp, endodontic treatment, as well as the status of the involved components of the dental complex.

The American Association of Endodontists classifies five specific variations of cracked teeth as follows: craze line, fractured cusp, cracked tooth, split tooth, and vertical root fracture [1]. For the purpose of diagnosis and treatment, attention must be given to the origin of pain since it can arise from any one or combination of the components of the dental complex such as just enamel, enamel extending to the E–D junction, enamel/dentin, enamel/dentin/pulp, as well as fractures that involve just the crown, just the root, as well as the extent of involvement of the periodontal ligament (PDL) and alveolus (tooth socket).

Another perplexing finding is that fractures may develop slowly or suddenly, and symptoms may change rapidly complicating a clear-cut clinical analysis. Radiographs may be helpful in determining the nature of a fracture but are not necessarily diagnostic in that they provide only a 2-dimensional image of a 3-dimensional problem. Computerized tomography (CT) is much more revealing but not practical for the general practitioner due to the cost of equipment.

Ellis defined an incomplete tooth fracture as a "fracture plane of unknown depth and direction passing through tooth structure that may advance and communicate with the pulp and/or periodontal ligament" [2]. However, symptoms will vary in accordance with the dental components affected. Thus, this definition does not lend itself to a distinct diagnosis and treatment.

Vertical fractures "involving the pulp" will not receive the in-depth attention that transverse fractures receive because they are usually readily identified and best resolved by extraction. On the other hand, transverse fractures including oblique

E. Lado, R. Caudle, *Pathway to Diagnosis and Management of Toothaches*,
https://doi.org/10.1007/978-3-031-75262-9_3

and horizontal fractures involving varying components of the dental complex account for an array of symptoms.

This chapter considers signs and symptoms likely to present from fractures involving specific parts of the dental complex. The proposed presentation uses a modified version of Kahler's 2008 Classification of Tooth Fractures [3].

3.2 Modified Classification of Coronal Fractures (Refer to Table 3.1)

Class I: Fractured Enamel only (Crazing)

Class II: Transverse fracture enamel & dentin not involving the Radicular PDL or pulp

Table 3.1 Tooth fracture classification and illustrations

	Associate Symptoms
Class I: Fractured enamel only (crazing) 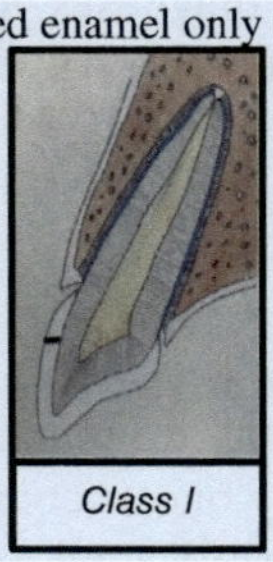	Stimulation of a-∂ fibers result in a sharp pain that returns to normal shortly upon removal of stimulus. Often not cusp specific
Class II: Transverse fracture enamel and dentin not involving the PDL or pulp 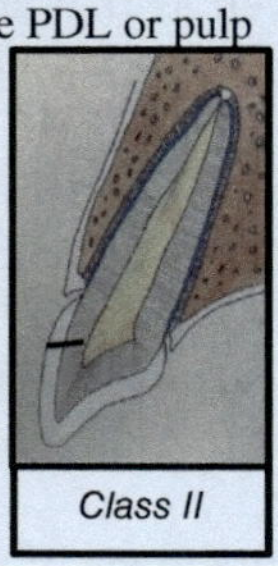	Sharp dental pain attributed to Brännström's theory of dentin hypersensitivity in response to mechanical or thermal stimulus of a-∂ fibers. Cusp specific
Class III: Transverse fracture involving the Pulp but not the PDL 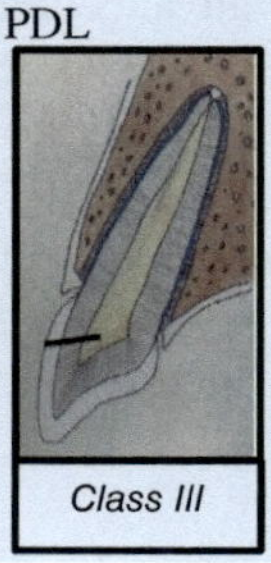	Symptoms vary in accordance with pulp status. Apical pathosis may be present. Not necessarily cusp specific. Initially sharp then aching pain as pulp dies

Table 3.1 (continued)

*Class II**: Transverse fracture involving the radicular PDL but not pulp 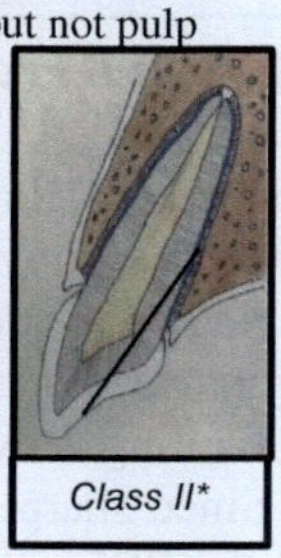	Sharp dentinal sensitivity to thermal and sharp tearing pain from PDL as broken cusp is displaced. Aching pain from PDL will prevail until attachment heals
*Class III**: Transverse fracture involving the pulp and the PDL 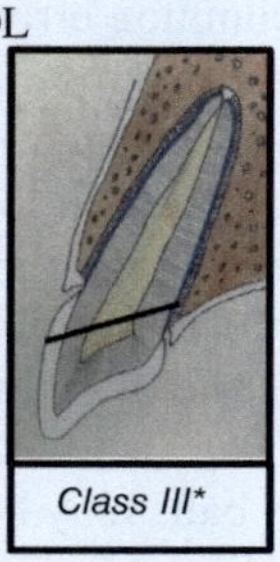	Symptoms vary in accordance with pulp status. Apical symptoms may present as well as PDL symptoms that are cusp specific
Class III(V): Vertical fracture through the pulp (not pictured)	Symptoms vary in accordance with pulp status Apical pathosis may present. Not necessarily cusp specific
Class IV (C) (R) (A): Root fractures 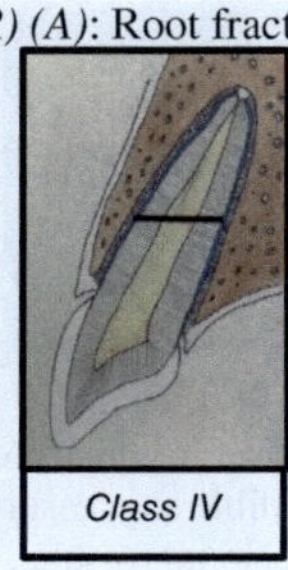	See next section on root fractures

Class II*: Transverse fracture involving the Radicular PDL but not pulp
Class III: Transverse fracture involving vital Pulp but not the PDL
Class III*: Transverse fracture involving vital Pulp and the PDL
Class III(V): Vertical fracture through the pulp

3.3 Classification of Root Fractures

Class IV(C): Transverse Root fracture @ cervical third (Cervical)
Class IV(R): Transverse Root fracture @ middle third (Radicular)

Class IV(A): Transverse Root fracture @ apical third (Apical)

3.4 Diagnosis: *Modified Classification of Coronal Fractures*

Fractured teeth may present diverse symptoms complicating diagnosis. Upon reviewing the modified classification, one can appreciate the array of symptoms triggered by involvement of the various components making up the dental complex. Besides the history and symptoms, a patient reports, diagnostic tests can help isolate the problem. Patients often present with a sharp pain upon biting. However, anytime tissue is torn, ripped, or lacerated, sharp pain ensues. Since sharp pain can arise from a-∂ fibers found in the dentinal tubules, pulp, and the PDL, appropriate tests must be conducted to determine the source of pain. A common error is to attribute "sharp pain" to a pulp problem when, in fact, it was arising from the PDL. This means the diagnostician must be able to reproduce the pain to determine the source.

A cursory exam with mirror and explorer may be sufficient to locate a fracture but may not reveal the extent to which each component of the tooth complex is involved. Unless the PDL is involved, there are no proprioceptive fibers stimulated. This makes it difficult for the patient to precisely locate the offending tooth. Tests involving occlusal forces may also stimulate the apical PDL but fail to identify the precise cusp causing the problem. Bite sticks and cotton balls may be used to identify the fractured cusp; however, a simple device (Tooth Slooth®) can deliver a precise force to each individual cusp duplicating the pain and facilitating confirmation of a fracture.

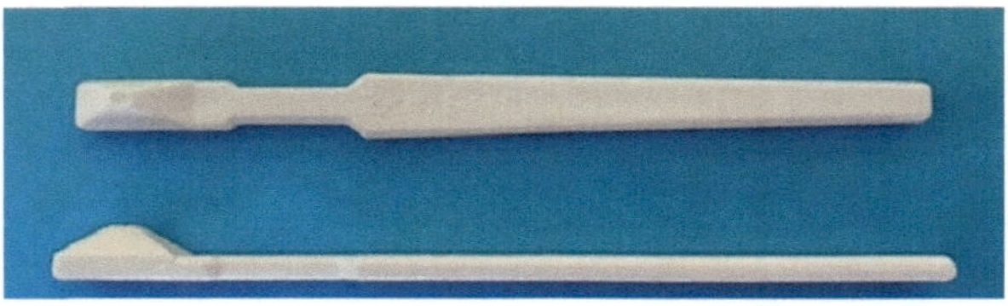

The dimple of the Tooth Slooth® should be placed on each cusp and a torquing force applied by the opposing teeth. This is done with a side-to-side motion of the mandible as pressure is applied. The force will spread the fractured cusp apart provoking pain. ® Professional Results, Inc. 17 Phaedra, Laguna Niguel, CA92677

Prior to using a Tooth Slooth, the "wiggle" test may provide sufficient information to identify a horizontal fracture. This consists of holding the crown with thumb and index fingers and wiggling it buccal-lingually, feeling for movement and crepitus as the separated segments rub against each other. A deeper radicular fracture may be better identified by feeling for root movement with one finger placed on the buccal bone and having the patient apply biting force to the suspect tooth and sliding their jaw side to side. The movement/vibration felt is known as "fremitus" and signals either a fractured or luxated tooth [4].

3.4.1 Class I: *Fractured (Enamel Only) (Crazing)*

Patients may complain of hypersensitivity to thermal challenges from teeth without a readily discernible pathosis; however, upon close inspection craze lines (hairlike surface cracks) may be seen in enamel. Since enamel is devoid of any sensory apparatus, fractures confined to enamel and not encroaching on the dentin-enamel junction (DEJ) will be asymptomatic. However, cracks that extend to the DEJ are likely to evoke a sharp pain to masticatory forces. Even thermal and chemical challenges can provoke an exaggerated sharp pain.

The tooth becomes sensitive to biting and/or releasing forces as forces at the DEJ alter the hydrodynamic pressures within the dental tubules containing odontogenic processes and exciting the a-∂ fibers that accompany them. This sensibility is consistent with Brännström's hydrodynamic theory of dentin hypersensitivity [5, 6] (see Addendum). It is presumed that pain results from distortion of the odontoblasts caused by movement of extracellular or intracellular fluid. These changes may be sufficient to provoke the a-∂ fibers.

An alternative suggestion is that pain caused by an enamel fracture is not necessarily due to an inflammatory reaction of the pulp provoked by cell death and the production of PgE_2 but likely result from repeated stimulation of the a-∂ nerve fibers accompanying the odontoblastic processes into the dentinal tubules resulting in allodynia. (An exaggerated pain to a non-noxious challenge, i.e., touch, chemical, or thermal/air, suggests an allodynia [7]. See discussion of allodynia in Chap. 1).

The patient may be adamant that a particular tooth is the culprit but with the absence of proprioceptive fibers in the pulp, the patient can be mistaken. It is reasonable to suspect that the symptoms suggest a symptomatic irreversible pulpitis (SIP) but in the absence of spontaneous pain, a more likely explanation is that the crazing has extended to the DEJ, acknowledged to be a highly sensitive area to touch, thermal and chemical challenges [8].

Mineral deposits and formation of reparative dentin can seal the tubules blocking stimulation of the a-∂ fibers and the pain wanes. Desensitizers such as Gluma® may be very helpful in reducing or completely eliminating the pain by sealing the outer portion of the tubule.

Chewing ice or a blow to the jaw can cause crazing of the enamel resulting in sensitivity. Parenthetically, a blow sufficiently forceful to compromise the blood supply to the pulp could also result in pulpitis and eventual necrosis of the pulp. Periodic evaluation of the pulp following trauma is appropriate. Brännström's theory no longer applies once the odontoblasts die via apoptosis (programmed cell death) and necrose [9]. Brännström's theory is only applicable to dentin housing odontogenic processes.

RCT or extraction will be necessary if the pain becomes spontaneous or the pulp dies. If the pulp remains healthy but pain persists some patients with crazed enamel resulting in "Dentinal Hypersensitivity" may opt for definitive treatment (full coverage or RCT and full coverage) just for relief. This scenario is likely if the pulp fails to wall off the area with tertiary (reparative) dentin. It is prudent to ensure all other proximal teeth and tissues are ruled out as the source of the pain prior to initiating irreversible treatment.

3.4.2 Class II: *Transverse Fracture Enamel and Dentin Not Involving the PDL or Pulp*

There is immediate pain as soon as dentin is involved with a fracture assuming the pulp and odontoblastic processes are viable. It is said that minute fractures hurt upon release of pressure. This axiom is not absolute and should not be pathognomonic of a "minute" fracture. (See prior discussion of crazed enamel)

When dentin is fractured, but not completely separated, biting forces cause the dentinal tubules to spread apart. Pain results from distortion of the remaining intact tubules changing the hydrodynamic pressure surrounding the odontoblastic processes [10]. When the applied force is removed (upon release), the fractured part returns to its original position again changing the hydrodynamic pressure resulting in pain. Since a-∂ sensory fibers accompany odontoblastic processes in the dentinal tubules the quality of reported pain upon biting should be "sharp" "shooting" and relatively short duration. A tooth, with exposed dentinal tubules but an intact pulp, will likely be sensitive to applied forces, thermal challenges, as well as caustic agents, but should not present with spontaneous or prolonged pain.

An occlusal force applied to the fractured cusp should elicit pain but painless when applied to the remaining cusps. On the other hand, thermal stimulation of the fractured portion may not be painful unless the challenge exerts a physical force against the fractured segment. This conundrum may be explained by the fact that it is only the broken cusp that moves and not the rest of the tooth. Since there is no movement of the intact portion of the tooth, there is no distortion of the dentinal tubules to cause pain. On the other hand, dentinal tubules that communicate with the pulp will likely respond to the thermal challenge. If forces applied to the uninvolved cusps of the suspect tooth cause pain, an inflammatory process involving the pulp, root, or apical PDL may be suspected and should be investigated.

Evidence of past fractured cusps not involving the pulp are commonly seen on maxillary premolars and lingual cusps of mandibular molars. Another cusp commonly fractured is the mesial buccal of the maxillary first molars. Patients will not report pain if mineral deposits have occluded the dentinal tubules and/or the pulp protected itself by laying down reparative dentin.

3.4.3 Class II*: *Transverse Fracture Involving the PDL But not Pulp*

If the fracture is completely through the dentin and extends through to the cementum and PDL, prostaglandins will be produced due to cellular death taking place within the PDL. This adds a periodontal component to the pain patients experience.

Recall C-fibers found in the PDL transmit an aching pain. The increase of PgE_2 from damaged cells lowers the pain threshold of the C-fibers; thus, it is common for the patient to experience a prolonged moderate aching discomfort arising from the PDL and not the pulp until the fractured part is removed and the area heals.

When a fracture extends into the PDL space, a lateral periodontal abscess may develop at the level of the fracture. It may even develop a sinus tract that could appear to originate from the apex of a tooth leading one to conclude the tooth has a chronic apical abscess (presence of a sinus tract). The origin of the abscess may be detected radiographically by tracing the sinus tract with a gutta-percha cone.

Keep in mind that when a transverse fracture (still attached to the PDL) is displaced a sharp "lancinating" pain will result as the fractured cusp tears at the PDL. This is not to be mistaken for pulpal pain from a-∂ fibers rather it is "neuropathic pain" caused by immediate injury to the nerve fibers. However, sharp pain to a thermal challenge may also arise from a-∂ fibers found in vital pulp.

If the fractured part is removed, the remaining exposed dentin may be sensitive to thermal, chemical, and mechanical challenges. Brännström's hydrodynamic theory will prevail until the odontoblasts die or tertiary dentin and/or mineral deposits seal the tubules. As previously noted, this scenario is evidenced by long-standing asymptomatic fractures of maxillary premolars and lingual cusps of the mandibular molars and mesial buccal cusps of maxillary first molars.

A common complaint following a complete fracture of a cusp (not involving the pulp) is the remaining sharp area of the remaining tooth structure irritating the tongue. These areas should be smoothed or temporally restored to prevent traumatic ulceration of proximal soft tissues (especially the tongue). Caution must be exercised when using acid etch composites on the newly exposed dentin. This can may eventually lead to death of the odontoblasts and a sterile necrosis of the pulp [11] (see Chap. 2).

Although most recent studies suggest that unless there is microleakage the use of etching and composites is safe, there is a dearth of controlled clinical studies confirming that pulpal health prevails over the long-term following the use of total-etch and resin-bonding techniques on dentin [12]. This author (EL) has encountered numerous teeth, restored with bonding materials, that pulps have subsequently become inflamed or necrosed, most of which were not pulp-capped but had prior amalgam restorations removed out of concern of mercury toxicity.

3.4.4 Class III: *Transverse Fracture Involving Vital Pulp But not the PDL*

It is not unusual for a simple enamel/dentinal fracture to encroach upon the pulp chamber. Symptoms are initially the same as mentioned above for a Class II fracture but once the fracture involves the pulp (Class III), and the pulp becomes inflamed, the initial sharp provoked pain is followed by a spontaneous prolonged aching pain that can vary with intensity as the pulp dies. This change is brought on by partial pulp necrosis increasing the levels of PgE_2 and lowering the pain threshold of the C-fibers located deeper in the canal. The further apically a coronal fracture extends, the greater the chance of pulp involvement.

It may take a few hours for the apex to become sensitive to percussion but until then, symptoms of just a symptomatic irreversible pulpitis (SIP) should prevail. As the pulp necroses, inflammatory mediators such as PgE_2 start to pass through the apex causing an inflammatory response, lowering the pain threshold at the apex, and the tooth becomes sensitive to percussion. This condition is referred to as symptomatic apical periodontitis (SAP). Note, an infection has yet to occupy the apical PDL.

Once bacteria proliferate at the apex, cells die and acute inflammatory cells accumulate in the area initiating the formation of an acute apical abscess (AAA). A constant aching pain will persist and swelling (edema) will likely follow. Once the abscess erodes through the cortical bone and periosteum, a fluctuant swelling (abscess) can develop. This swelling usually occurs in the vestibular region but can find its way to a fascial space resulting in a life-threatening infection. In time, a sinus tract may develop allowing pus to drain and provide temporary relief.

AAEs' diagnostic paradigm classifies development of a sinus tract as a chronic apical abscess (CAA). An open pulp canal can act similarly to a sinus tract and the pain subsides similarly to the CAA.

If the purulence is draining through the canal, any attempt to seal the canal with a temporary restoration will likely precipitate pain and cause the abscess to seek a path of least resistance, i.e., a fascial space. A common means of preventing a space infection is to establish drainage by I&D, thereby providing an easy path for the abscess to drain. Systemic antibiotics would be appropriate along with close follow-up.

3.4.5 Class III*: *Transverse Fracture Involving the Pulp and the PDL*

Once the class III fracture reaches the radicular PDL, any lateral displacement of the fractured cusp will provoke a sharp pain. This is especially noteworthy from a tooth with a non-vital pulp (i.e., necrotic or endotreated pulp by mimicking the sharp pain associated with an irreversible pulpitis).

3.4.6 Class III(V): *Vertical Fracture through the Pulp*

Vertical root fractures, usually seen in multi-rooted teeth, are longitudinally orientated mesial-distal and extend from the pulp chamber to the periodontium [13].

Symptoms vary initially from symptomatic irreversible pulpitis to a necrotic pulp with an apical abscess depending on the duration and course of the fracture. Most abscesses will manifest at the apex while some may be found at the furcation of multi-rooted teeth or the lateral portion of the root pending the course of the fracture. Usually, all cusps will respond with pain to masticatory forces. Restoration is rarely possible, and extraction is the treatment of choice.

3.5 Classification of Root Fractures (Refer to Diagram 3.1)

Traditionally, root fractures have been classified according to the location of the fracture and specifically whether it is located at the apical, middle, or coronal third of the root [14] (see Diagram 3.1). This classification is useful because the management and prognosis for root fractures vary according to location. The more apical horizontal fractures involving healthy pulps generally require the least management and have the best prognosis whereas coronal root fractures require the most complex management and have the worst prognosis. A major factor causing the poor prognosis is the propensity of bacterial infection due to exposure to oral flora calling for a more aggressive approach (endo, post, full coverage) to managing supracrestal root fractures than what is usually required for middle and apical fractures.

The prognosis of a mid- and apical root fracture of a "healthy pulp" is better than coronal root fractures and underscores the recommendation to not remove the pulp as part of the emergency management. Instead, a "wait and see" approach should be taken in order to monitor the tooth to see if signs of pulp death develop. These teeth can always have root canal treatment done at a later time when a definitive diagnosis of pulp necrosis and infection has been made. There is no advantage, and no evidence or sense, in commencing root canal treatment early or as a "preventive measure." Such an approach is contraindicated because it removes the most important tissue (the dental pulp), which can provide the best healing outcomes (i.e., internal repair with hard tissue). Pulp survival is dependent on the age of the patient at the time of the fracture with younger teeth having a better prognosis. This is because of the better vascularity and wider root canals assisting pulp revascularization at the fracture site.

Diagram 3.1 Image depicting root fractures

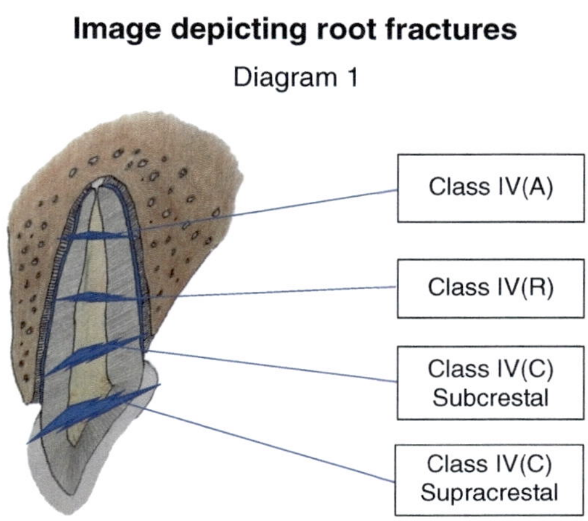

3.5.1 Class IV(C): *Transverse Root Fracture @ Coronal Third (Coronal)*

As can be seen in Table 3.1, the 10-year tooth loss for teeth with cervical fractures was 31.2%. Contrary to the more apically located fractures, the crown is usually lost due to the minimal attachment to the alveolus leaving the pulp in direct contact with the oral flora. Management and prognosis of coronal fractures invariably require RCT and post/core buildup for restoration. An alternative was implant or extraction.

There are several reasons for this failure rate. One major reason is that the pulp in crestal fractures is exposed to oral flora and more likely to become infected if untreated. Difficulty establishing a margin and the crown to root ratio may also hinder restoration.

Another possibility is that trauma is believed to trigger cervical resorption, especially if a bleaching procedure was performed [15]. It is reasonable to assume a tooth that has had the crown fractured off experienced some type of trauma and therefore is at risk of cervical resorption [16].

3.5.2 Class IV(R): *Transverse Root Fracture @ Middle Third (Radicular)*

Radicular fractures have a 10-year failure rate of 8.7%, significantly less than for a cervical fracture. The major difference between a cervical and mid- and apical root fractures is a lack of bacterial contamination of the pulp.

Contamination of the wound is unlikely *so long as the crown is not displaced*, and the pulp is not severed and was healthy prior to the fracture. Given this assumption odontoblasts in the pulp canal have favorable conditions to produce reparative dentin and reunite the apical and coronal fragments. It is a similar process to the formation of a dentinal bridge, except the dentin typically forms vertically along the canal walls at the fracture line rather than horizontally across the pulp space, it acts like a bone callus that stabilizes the fracture. The tooth needs splinting for 2–3 months to allow a dentinal callus to form [17].

So long as the pulp and alveolus heal, the symptoms will be transient and characteristic of mild aching pain. The crown may exhibit a reversible pulpitis until the inflammation in the pulp resolves and pulp heals. If the level of pulp pain increases, the remaining pulp is most likely necrosing and RCT may be attempted if a callus has formed uniting the two fragments.

On the other hand, swelling or increased aching pain signals the development of an abscess requiring extraction of the remaining tooth fragments.

3.5.3 Class IV(A): *Transverse Root Fracture @ Apical Third (Apical)*

Apical fractures present the lowest percent (7.7%) of fracture failures. However, if the force of the trauma compromises the blood supply to the pulp RCT is an option so long as the crown to root ratio is favorable. Otherwise, a conservative approach of waiting and watching is optimal. The tooth should be monitored (EPT and thermal tests) for several weeks and if symptoms arise, RCT should be considered.

A blow resulting in an apical fracture will often be sufficient to compromise the blood supply to the pulp, eventually causing pulp necrosis. Initially, a symptomatic irreversible pulpitis will soon result in a necrotic pulp. If RCT is the preferred treatment, an apicoectomy to remove the fractured remaining root tip may be warranted.

The following table is a summary of the data from the dental trauma guide website showing long-term outcomes for teeth with transverse root fractures. It shows that over a 10-year period 31% of teeth with fractures of the coronal third were lost over 10 years, whereas only 8.7% of teeth with mid-root fractures were lost over the same period of time [18].

	Number of years follow-up	Coronal 3rd root fracture	Middle 3rd root fracture	Apical 3rd root fracture
Total # of teeth		**16**	**46**	**13**
Teeth lost by years	**1**	*1*	2	*0*
	3	*1*	*3*	*1*
	10	5 **(31.2%)**	4 **(8.7%)**	**1 (7.7%)**
Pulp necrosis and infection of the root canal system	**1**	*5*	*12*	2
	3	*5*	*14*	*3*
	10	5	14	3
Pulp canal calcifications	**1**	2	*16*	2
	3	*4*	*24*	*5*
	10	*9*	*25*	*9*

The significance of this finding is that the prognosis of endodontic treatment is better with a horizontal fracture as the level approaches the apex.

Note: Numbers are cumulative over the follow-up periods of 1, 3, and 10 years. Adopted from: Abbott PV. Diagnosis and management of transverse root fractures. Dent Traumatol. 2019; 35:333-347

3.6 Conclusion

Although tooth fractures often present a diagnostic dilemma, appreciation for the various conditions sign and symptoms will allow for a focused process directing a diagnosis and subsequent treatment.

Abbott concluded: "Teeth with horizontal, oblique, or transverse root fractures have a very good long-term prognosis if the fracture is located in the apical to middle third of the root or if a horizontal fracture is located subcrestal in the coronal third of the root…with immediate repositioning and stabilization of the coronal portion…" However, "Supracrestal root fractures are the most difficult to manage and usually require removal of the coronal fragment, root canal treatment of the remaining root, and restoration."

References

1. Torabinejad M, Walton RE. Principles and practice of endodontics. 4th ed. Philadelphia: W.B. Saunders; 2002. p. 108–28.
2. Ellis SGS. Incomplete tooth fracture-proposal for a new definition. Br Dent J. 2001;190(8):424–8. https://doi.org/10.1038/sj.bdj.4800992.
3. Kahler W. The cracked tooth conundrum: terminology, classification, diagnosis and management. Am J Dent. 2008;21(5):275–82.
4. http://www.dent-wiki.com/foundations_of_periodontics/tooth-mobility-and-fremitus/.
5. Garberoglio R, Brännström M. Scanning electron microscopic investigation of human dentinal tubules. Arch Oral Biol. 1976;21(6):355–62. https://doi.org/10.1016/s0003-9969(76)80003-9.
6. West NX, Lussi A, Seong J, Hellwig E. Dentin hypersensitivity: pain mechanisms and aetiology of exposed cervical dentin. Clin Oral Investig. 2013;17(Suppl 1):S9–19. https://doi.org/10.1007/s00784-012-0887-x. Epub 2012 Dec 9.
7. Renton T, Wilson NH. Understanding and managing dental and orofacial pain in general practice. Br J Gen Pract. 2016;66(646):236–7. https://doi.org/10.3399/bjgp16X684901. PMID: 27127274; PMCID: PMC4838424.
8. Cohen JS, Reader A, Fertel R, Beck M, Meyers WJ. A radioimmunoassay determination of the concentrations of prostaglandins E2 and F2alpha in painful and asymptomatic human dental pulps. J Endod. 1985;11(8):330–5. https://doi.org/10.1016/s0099-2399(85)80039-x.
9. Mitsiadis TA, Feki A, Papaccio G, Catón J. Dental pulp stem cells, niches, and notch signaling in tooth injury. Adv Dent Res. 2011;23(3):275–9. https://doi.org/10.1177/0022034511405386.
10. Dionysopoulos D, Gerasimidou O, Beltes C. Dentin hypersensitivity: etiology, diagnosis and contemporary therapeutic approaches—a review in literature. Appl Sci. 2023;13(21):11632. https://doi.org/10.3390/app132111632.
11. Accorinte ML, Loguercio AD, Reis A, Muench A, de Araújo VC. Adverse effects of human pulps after direct pulp capping with the different components from a total-etch, three-step adhesive system. Dent Mater. 2005;21(7):599–607. https://doi.org/10.1016/j.dental.2004.08.008.
12. Bergenholtz G. Evidence for bacterial causation of adverse pulpal responses in resin-based dental restorations. Crit Rev Oral Biol Med. 2000;11(4):467–80. https://doi.org/10.1177/10454411000110040501.
13. Pitts DL, Natkin E. Diagnosis and treatment of vertical root fractures. J Endod. 1983;9(8):338–46. https://doi.org/10.1016/S0099-2399(83)80150-2.
14. Abbott PV. Diagnosis and management of transverse root fractures. Dent Traumatol. 2019;35(6):333–47. https://doi.org/10.1111/edt.12482.
15. Lado EA, Stanley HR, Weisman MI. Cervical resorption in bleached teeth. Oral Surg Oral Med Oral Pathol. 1983;55(1):78–80. https://doi.org/10.1016/0030-4220(83)90310-9.
16. Heithersay GS. Invasive cervical resorption following trauma. Aust Endod J. 1999;25(2):79–85. https://doi.org/10.1111/j.1747-4477.1999.tb00094.x.
17. Çiçek E, Yılmaz N, Koçak MM. Intraradicular splinting with endodontic instrument of horizontal root fracture. Case Rep Dent. 2015;2015:505370. https://doi.org/10.1155/2015/505370. Epub 2015 Jan 12. PMID: 25648395; PMCID: PMC4306357.
18. Abbott PV. Diagnosis and management of transverse root fractures. Dent Traumatol. 2019;35(6):333–47. https://doi.org/10.1111/edt.12482. Epub 2019 Oct 16.

Further Reading

Bourguignon C, Cohenca N, Lauridsen E, et al. International Association of Dental Traumatology guidelines for the management of traumatic dental injuries: 1. Fractures and luxations. Dent Traumatol. 2020;36(4):314–30.

Diagnostic Testing

4

4.1 Introduction

When diagnosing a toothache, the attendant pain must be assigned to specific components of the dental complex based on the history, clinical signs, symptoms, and test results that are consistent with the chief complaint (CC). Several "diagnostic tests" are available to assess the source of dental pain. Information gained from each test helps direct the diagnostician to the source of the pain as well as the diagnosis. The following discussion addresses methods of conducting tests as well as interpretation of the information obtained.

NOTE: A thorough evaluation of your patients' medical history and vitals MUST BE completed prior to initiating invasive diagnostic procedures.

4.2 Diagnostic Tests

4.2.1 Sensorial Examination

A cursory visual inspection of the patients' extraoral features may reveal swelling, redness, and/or other abnormalities related to the chief complaint. Note any asymmetries or deformities including a loss of function. Following the extraoral examination, the intraoral examination should consist of an inspection of the hard and soft tissues of the oral cavity including the posterior and lateral borders of the tongue, vestibule, palate, and post-pharyngeal area. Look for signs of pathosis including changes in texture, color, swelling, ulceration, hemorrhage, sinus tracts, purulence, etc. When examining the dentition, look for: caries, evidence of erosion, abrasion, attrition, trauma (fractures/discoloration), extensive and or defective restorations, food impactions, appearance of the gingiva, exudate, plaque, calculus, etc., and

E. Lado, R. Caudle, *Pathway to Diagnosis and Management of Toothaches*,
https://doi.org/10.1007/978-3-031-75262-9_4

connect the findings to the chief complaint. Obvious conditions may be adequately diagnosed without further testing, such as an exposed pulp chamber or a pulp polyp. One means of evaluation is lost with the use of masks and that is the sense of smell. Ketone or putrid breath could be a sign of systemic disease or the foul odor of necrotic tissue as in ANUG.

All too frequently a problem is obscured that requires further testing or biopsy. Diagnostic tests should be dictated by the prevailing signs and symptoms and unnecessary testing should be avoided, such as conducting a thermal test on a partially impacted third molar with a pericoronitis and no visible caries. (Every toothache is not pulpal in origin.)

4.2.2 Transillumination

It is possible to detect abnormalities by directing a high-intensity light through hard or soft tissues. Hard tissue abnormalities including interproximal caries and tooth fractures may be detected. Soft tissue abnormalities including foreign bodies and variations in tissue density may also be identified. Transillumination can even reveal a congested sinus, especially should the patient complain of pressure pain over the eye consistent with frontal sinusitis.

4.2.3 Palpation

This test is applicable to both extraoral and intraoral examination. Tenderness to palpation is a strong indicator that something is wrong even without the presence of swelling. However, the appearance of indurated or fluctuant swollen area in close proximity to teeth suggests cellulitis or abscess. An abscess in soft tissue will be fluctuant and tender to touch. Palpation may express pus from a sinus tract or the gingival sulcus that might otherwise go unnoticed. Swelling that has increased slowly over weeks or months requires further evaluation to rule out a tumor. Hard swelling is an indication that the abscess has yet to break through the periosteum or an expansile lesion suggesting a cyst of neoplasm. Alternately, an external, firm, indurated, swelling that occurred within hours may well be a collection of edematous fluids (cellulitis).

Local infiltration anesthesia may be intolerable or ineffectual when a cellulitis is present at the chosen site of injection, but a course of an antibiotic and time should allow an abscess to coalesce, and effectiveness of local anesthesia will improve, enabling I&D or extraction with minimal discomfort. A nerve block may be attempted if the swelling is not in the injection site.

In the meantime, a course of antibiotics and an anti-inflammatory (if not contraindicated) should provide some relief. It is important that the patient stay hydrated and consume nutrients such as found in supplement drinks if eating regular food is impaired. The patient should be advised not to place warmth on the outside of the swelling, warm intraoral rinses are encouraged so that an abscess is drawn intraoral and not on the outer surface of the dermis.

4.2.4 Percussion

The status of the apical periodontal ligament may be evaluated by gently tapping the cusps of teeth with the blunt end of a metal instrument. Tenderness to apically directed percussion is suggestive of symptomatic apical periodontitis (SAP).

NOTE: Inflammation is the body's response to repair injured/damaged tissue such as seen with bruxing or trauma. It does not necessarily signal an infection within the dental complex. Thus, a tooth may present with Symptomatic Apical Periodontitis (SAP) totally unrelated to an infection. Use of an antibiotic is not indicated unless there is evidence of an infection.

On the other hand, a pulpal abscess confined to the pulp chamber may send PgE_2 to the apical periodontium lowering the pain threshold of the C-fibers resulting in SAP. Until the tooth becomes sensitive to palpation or depressible in the socket, it is not likely the pulp abscess has progressed into the PDL through the apex. Although percussion is not an appropriate test to evaluate the status of pulp tissue, it can lead to identifying the tooth causing the chief complaint. It could also direct you to consider a fractured tooth. In the case of a fractured cusp usually just the involved cusps are symptomatic to occlusal forces unless the fracture also involves the pulp. Sensitivity to percussion can also be caused by traumatic occlusion, bruxism, or even a non-dental condition such as sinusitis or trigeminal neuralgia.

When performing this test, first percuss several teeth away from the suspected tooth and work toward it. Lightly tapping the cusps overlying each root three times in rapid succession (Tap, Tap, Tap) repeat on next cusp/tooth and ask the patient to indicate by raising their hand when it feels "different" from the rest or mimics the pain associated with their CC.

This process should be done with minimal hesitation between cusps and teeth. Do not stop to ask, "did that hurt?" The patient's wincing or withdrawal reaction as the test is conducted usually conveys all you need to know. This is one reason that tapping should be done gently. Firm rapping will prime the patients' avoidance reaction making it difficult to read the patients' reaction.

Testing may start with teeth on the contralateral side and work toward the suspect tooth to establish the patient's base line reaction. Start at least 3 teeth away from the suspect tooth. Testing just one "control" tooth and comparing the result with the suspect tooth does not establish a baseline reaction. Once the offending tooth is challenged the patient often indicates "That's it."

You should not stop there but continue percussing beyond the suspect tooth to be sure that the offending tooth is identified. Pain often radiates from the affected area and teeth adjacent to the offender may also prove sensitive. If the patient is not sure which tooth hurts the most or if you are unable to elicit a reaction, repeat the challenge again asking the patient to single out the most sensitive one. (Which one bothers your more… #1) …Tap Tap Tap (or #2) Tap Tap Tap.

The patient may be experiencing referred pain so if they fail to identify the offending tooth in one arch be sure to rule out referred pain from teeth in the opposing arch. Also consider the possibility of referred pain from other major systems including the heart or other conditions such as myofascial pain or neurological problems including "trigeminal neuralgia."

The patient will often wince or recoil when the suspect tooth is percussed, confirming their subjective account of the chief complaint. Do not ask the patient to identify the tooth that "hurts" since pain is very subjective, ask them to let you know when the tooth that "feels different" from the rest is percussed. Their reaction will let you know if it hurts. Be sure to lightly percuss each cusp overlying the roots of multi-rooted teeth and to move methodically from one tooth to the next allowing sufficient time for the patient to respond.

When healthy teeth are percussed, you should notice a sharp crisp sound. Periodically you will encounter a tooth that elicits a characteristic "thud" sound. This sound may indicate an inflammatory reaction in the PDL. However, it is not pathognomonic of apical periodontitis due to an inflamed pulp since a cracked tooth, one in hyper-occlusion, a heavily restored tooth, or even tapping enamel undermined by caries may yield a similar sound.

4.2.5 Mobility

Mobility is best determined by applying lateral and occlusal forces to a tooth and observing the extent of tooth movement. Class 1 < 1 mm) and Class 2 (> 1 mm) lateral movement may indicate a loss of periodontal support and/or occlusal trauma, whereas Class 3 (apical mobility) usually indicates the presence of an apical abscess.

Fremitus is a common method of detecting mobility. It is accomplished by placing a finger on the labial/buccal alveolus and having the patient apply an occlusal force by biting with side-to-side movement. If movement is felt, it may indicate a tooth in hyper-occlusion, or advanced periodontal bone loss. It may also present if there is a horizontal fracture. Moving a tooth with a fractured root may yield crepitus (crackling sound/sensation) as the divided parts of the tooth grind against each other.

4.2.6 Periodontal Probing

Another important method of evaluating the health of the periodontium is to do a thorough probing of the gingival attachments. Periodontal defects greater than 3 mm and/or furcation involvements should be noted. While probing, look for the presence of local factors, such as excess bleeding, suppuration, food impactions, calculus, overhangs, open margins, sinus tracks, and pseudo-pockets associated with erupting teeth.

4.2.7 Pulp Testing

4.2.7.1 Thermal

The fact that sudden exaggerated temperature changes may cause tooth pain is a well-observed phenomenon. Brännström proposed that thermal changes cause a distortion of the fluid within dentinal tubules that mechanically stimulates sensory nerve endings resulting in pain [1, 2]. Once the pressure from the fluid stabilizes, the pain subsides.

Van Hassel has pointed out that normal teeth may initially respond painfully to cold stimulus, but if the cold stimulus is held in place long enough the pain will dissipate. He proposed the coefficient of expansion of dentin fluid is estimated to be approximately ten times greater than that of the tubule wall, therefore the shape of the odontoblast could accommodate the change in the applied forces with time and the pain subsides [3]

Brännström's theory only applies to dentinal pain. However, an inflamed pulp also responds to thermal changes and the mechanism of pulp pain is contingent on the degree of inflammation and levels of PgE_2. If the cold source is held in place, the pain may also subside but for a different reason.

I would argue that relief comes from cold decreasing the accumulation of fluids (edema) and blood flow within the pulp tissues reducing pressure within the confines of the pulp chamber and canal and thereby reducing stimulation of the a-∂ and C-fibers. If the reduction were only within the dentinal tubules, the patient would still have pain from the vital pulp. I suggest that relief would be provided not only from the sharp shooting pain conducted by the a-∂ fibers found within the tubules but also the aching pain from C-fibers in the inflamed pulp. This speculation is consistent with the concept of applying ice to a traumatic injury to reduce swelling.

Recall from the discussion in the section "Diagnosis of Odontogenic Pain" (Chap. 1) thermal (cold) challenge provoked the a-∂ fibers (terminating in the dentinal tubules and coronal pulp) resulting in a short duration sharp pain alerting the tooth of an external assault but it was the C-fibers that provoked a long duration aching pain as their cell membranes are lysed and arachidonic acid is converted to PgE_2.

The presumption that if the aching pain provoked by the thermal stimulus is prolonged then the C-fibers in the pulp would be affected, suggesting the pulp incapable of self-repair due to the amount of cellular death taking place.

As such, there is a tendency to assign a diagnosis of symptomatic irreversible pulpitis (SIP) to any tooth that exhibits pain to a thermal challenge for longer than 10 seconds. The converse is not valid since we know some normal teeth especially with partially necrotic pulps may not respond to thermal challenges simply because the remaining vital tissue is out of the range of the temperature change.

We also see teeth diagnosed with an inflamed pulp that exhibit an allodynia not an irreversible pulpitis. The distinguishing feature is that an inflamed pulp will have spontaneous pain along with a prolonged hyper-response, whereas the tooth with allodynia will have a heightened response to a stimulus without prolonged or spontaneous pain.

Teeth undergoing orthodontic movement, vital bleaching, acid etching, or even neighboring teeth with their apex in close proximity to an inflamed sinusitis may all temporarily exhibit prolonged thermal hypersensitivity [4, 5]. This should not be interpreted as an allodynia rather pain radiating from a proximal source of inflammation.

A very high percentage of teeth affected by "irreversible" pulpitis react positively to thermal challenges with prolonged and more intense pain. But not all irreversible pulpitis pulps will respond similarly. It has been estimated that 20% of normal teeth do not response to thermal challenges. The presence of tertiary dentin could account for a good portion of this 20% as could teeth with partial pulp necrosis. When this occurs, electric pulp testing may help in determining if the pulp is still vital. No response to an EPT can signal a partial pulp necrosis breaking the circuit. Teeth with a significant amount of reparative dentin may also impede the flow of current.

A "control" tooth is suggested when performing diagnostic tests to establish a base line reaction from the patient. (The use of a "control" tooth is addressed in the addendum and begs your attention.) Prior to actually testing the suspect tooth, a question needs answering and that is: What information is gained by testing a "control tooth"? And what criteria determines the selection of the control tooth? Calling into question, is it truly a control?

If the patient is complaining of spontaneous *pulpal* pain or has had to resort to analgesics to quell the pain, the question of reversible vs irreversible is moot. The fact that a patient complains of unprovoked/spontaneous pulpal pain answers that question. If the patient complains of provoked pain of short duration, only the objective of testing is to identify the offending tooth. In some circumstances, the reason for the chief complaint is obvious; it is the obtuse diagnosis that stumps us.

Since proprioceptive fibers are not present in pulp tissue, the patient may have difficulty locating the source of pain. This is often the case involving heavily restored or fractured teeth where the apical periodontium is not involved. This presents a conundrum difficulty identifying the offending tooth makes it difficult to select a contralateral tooth with similar characteristics to use as a control.

I suggest testing several normal appearing teeth with cold, *before* testing the suspected tooth, to establish the basic response pattern of the patient. Testing other teeth away from the suspect tooth first should not increase their apprehension and thus their responses should be more reliable. This holds true for most diagnostic tests except the EPT.

My suggestion is to test several (4, 5) teeth away from and moving slowly but deliberately toward the suspected offender (using teeth cross arch is acceptable.) Keep the cold challenge on the tooth for a couple of seconds after they indicate sensibility. Wait for the patients' response to indicate it has dissipated before proceeding to the next tooth in line. Eventually, the patient may respond to the offending tooth by recoiling or crying out "That's it."

In performing thermal tests have the patient note the intensity as well as the quality and duration of the elicited pain. Once the painful tooth is found instruct the patient to signal with their hand (**1**) **Up.** When they first feel discomfort. Then remove the challenge. (**2**) **Down** When it goes away, (3) Then ask them **to describe any difference** in sensation felt between the suspect tooth as compared to baseline teeth and if there was any lingering pain and how long it lasted. This information can then be assimilated and processed to arrive at a diagnosis.

Cold Tests

An aerosolized coolant (Endo-Ice®) is commonly used for cold tests. When sprayed on a cotton pellet, ice crystals form from moisture in the ambient air. Do not rush to place the pellet on the tooth, rather allow a few seconds and witness the ice crystals form. Once crystals begin to form, place the pellet on enamel that is supported by sound dentin. Failure to do so may result in a flawed test because a restoration, caries, or a void could insulate the pulp from the thermal challenge. Alternatively, the dentin may become so cold as to transmit the change in temperature to the PDL fibers and confound a test result.

When supported enamel is not available due to caries, an alternative to an ice test is to blow a gentle stream of air from an air syringe into the cavity. Keep the stream going for a few seconds in an attempt to provoke the pulp. This is not to test the dentin rather to stimulate a reaction from the pulp that mimics the CC.

A prolonged reaction to a thermal challenge may indicate an irreversible pulpitis but is not pathognomonic. On the other hand, if the patient has complained of spontaneous pain, the prolonged reaction to cold suggests symptomatic irreversible pulpitis. Bleached teeth, bruxed teeth, teeth near an inflamed sinus may respond with a prolonged sensitivity to thermal stimulus but should not have had spontaneous pain. The most important symptom suggestive of an irreversible pulpitis is "Spontaneous Pulpal Pain." This pain originates from PgE_2 lowering the pain threshold of C-fibers. It should have an aching quality and possibly throb (pulsate). Duration of pain is not pathognomonic for irreversible pulpitis, although we tend to diagnose the condition as reversible if the pain is less than 10 seconds. The short duration may be the result of an inadequate change in temperature to provoke a full reaction.

Depending on the change in temperature transferred the duration of the reaction time could vary. So, it is necessary to keep the test in place long enough to provoke a valid reaction. Patients that report pain to cold may shorten the time of the test by indicating they feel it, thereby avoiding the anticipated pain interrupting the test and indicating the pain was of short duration not prolonged reaction that would have suggested an irreversible pulpitis. The fact that a patient complains of having been wakened by the pain or has had to take OTC analgesics is a much more reliable in formulating the diagnosis as opposed to a thermal test.

The main reason to conduct thermal testing is to identify the offending tooth as well as confirm symptoms provided by the patient and to rule out referred pain from another tooth.

Sometimes the patient will report relief during one of the diagnostic tests. Remember, teeth failing to react to thermal stimulation may yet have vital pulps, but this does not confirm that the pulps are healthy. In fact, the coronal portion of the pulp chamber could be void of tissue with vital pulp remaining further apical in the canal. Such a tooth may not respond to thermal challenge nor test "vital" with the EPT.

If a sealed tooth has a void in the pulp chamber, but vital pulp tissue remains in the canal, thermal changes can affect the pressure within the hollow chamber (see discussion of Aerodontalgia page 36–37) considering "Combined Gas Laws" specifically "Charles Law" that expresses a relation between pressure to temperature.

Heat Tests

Heat tests can be carried out with dental "green stick molding compound"[1] by the following technique. Place one end of the stick near a heat source. As the heat softens the material, it will begin to bend from its own weight. While holding the compound with one hand mold the softened end to a blunted point with your gloved fingers. Prior to molding be sure to coat your gloved fingers with petroleum jelly. My personal preference is the green stick which gives a prolonged working time without dripping. This will not only prevent you from burning yourself or the patient, but it will also temper the outside of the stick compound preventing it from sticking to the tooth or dripping on the patient as you move toward the suspect tooth.

Place the thermal challenge on sound tooth structure avoiding any restoration or the gingiva. The stick compound provides a controlled, safe heat. This is not true with heated metallic instruments because the temperature of the metal that meets the tooth surface cannot be controlled.

When performing thermal tests, several proximal teeth are tested first working toward the suspect tooth. The patient is asked to signal by raising their hand when "Let me know when you feel it and when the sensation goes away." Heat tests are indicated to identify the tooth responsible for a chief complaint of heat-provoking tooth pain. That is, if the patient complains about heat causing pain, duplicate it with the heat test.

4.2.7.2 Electric Pulp Testing

When diagnosing a toothache, it is often necessary to establish the overall health of the dental pulp [6]. The EPT has historically been considered a "vitality" test. Unfortunately, it has limitations and results are subject to misinterpretation. It has recently been disregarded by many diagnosticians because it was shown to be less accurate in determining vitality than thermal testing. However, it is a valuable adjunct when used in conjunction with thermal testing [7]. If used skillfully and results properly interpreted, the EPT can be of value in some cases where thermal tests are inconclusive. NOTE: It is not a substitute for a thermal test!

It is well established there is no correlation between EPT readings and actual pulpal health. The EPT is a "continuity tester" not a "vitality" tester, calling into question the studies comparing results to thermal tests [8]. The actual voltage is dependent on the resistance/impedance and current density within the circuit (a definition of current density follows.)

Healthy teeth sometimes yield EPT readings that vary considerably from those of similar teeth in the same mouth and even on the same tooth from 1 day to another. Comparing readings from a contralateral "control tooth" is not warranted since the digital readouts are an ordinal scale not affixed to an actual voltage, not to mention the myriad of factors can affect the test readings [9].

The Analytic Technology® pulp tester is designed so that voltage gradually increases to avoid shocking the patient. It will reset to zero automatically a few

---

[1] Working temperatures of Kerr compound sticks are: Green 122–124° F; Gray: 130° F; Red: 130–132° F Check working temps for other manufactures.

seconds after removal from the tooth. This prevents an accidental high-voltage shock to the tooth and ample time to observe the digital reading. This was a problem with the older analog pulp testers. When contact was lost, the tendency was to replace the tester forgetting to reset the rheostat and delivering high voltage to the tooth. Consequently, many dentists avoided its use, often at the patients' insistence.

In order to use a pulp tester successfully, there are several important steps that must be followed. First, clean, "air-dry," and isolate the tooth in question. Adjust the dial that controls the rate voltage increases between 4 and 6; apply a little toothpaste (electrolyte) to the EPT probe tip and place the probe tip (on enamel supported by viable dentin) preferably between the middle and gingival third of the clinical crown. This location is preferred since it is most likely to have intact dentinal tubules allowing the electric charge travel to the pulp.

Avoid contact with the gingiva or any restorations as inadvertent contact may short circuit and cause a false reading or an unwanted shock. Once the probe tip is stabilized on the tooth, instruct the patient to reach up and gently grasp the probe handle and hold it until they feel a "pulsing or tingling sensation." This will complete the circuit allowing an electric charge to flow with voltage increasing incrementally. Once sensation is felt, the patient is instructed to release the probe handle breaking the circuit. The display remains on for a few seconds allowing ample time to be read.

The need to test a control tooth is questionable in that if a control tooth is tested first, it will alert the patient to be guarded against a shock applied to the already painful tooth. And if it is applied to a contralateral tooth after testing the suspect tooth, it delivers an unnecessary shock since the desired information has already been obtained. The rub comes in the interpretation of the findings. Key concepts to consider are available in the "helpful hints" that follow at the end of this section.

Current Density

A major reason the EPT has fallen from grace as a diagnostic aid is a failure to appreciate the concept of current density. Current density (J) is the amount of electric current (EC) per unit time that flows through a unit area of a chosen cross section. Recall the formula $E = IR$, where E is the electro-motive force (volts), I is the current (amps per unit time), and R is resistance (ohms).

The pulp tester attempts to maintain a constant low amperage (I) while the voltage (E) is proportional to the resistance (R). A high resistance calls for a high voltage to maintain the flow of EC.

More force is required to "push" the current through a small opening than through a large one.

Current density (J) is calculated by amperes/area in m^2 or $J = I/A$ where amperage (I) is the number of coulombs moving past a given point in 1 s and A is the area in meters squared.

In this case, current density is the concentration of electricity flowing through a restricted area (the tooth apex). According to "Pouillet's Law," resistance is inversely proportional to the cross-sectional area [10]. Applying this concept to the tooth, we see that voltage must increase to overcome the resistance as the size of the apex decreases. Thus, the smaller the apex, the greater the force (volts) required to push the EC through the apex and patients feel the electric stimulus once the EC reaches the threshold potential of the sensory nerves.

Since the physics of fluid flowing through a pipe is analogous to the flow of electricity, the following comparison is offered. Picture the force of five gallons of water per minute coming out of a storm drain. You could imagine a small animal drinking from such a drain quite comfortably.

Now imagine the same five gallons per minute flowing out of an oral hygiene irrigating device. That much water forced through the small opening of the device may be sufficient to tear the gingiva from the bone. Restricting the diameter of the opening increases resistance and therefore the force required to drive the water through the point of exit.

This concept applies to the flow of electricity through the tooth. Because the current flows through the pulp tissues and out through the apex, a large apex presents a low current density, allowing current to flow with little force (volts), the way water flows through a storm drain. If the EC does not reach, the threshold potential of the nerves it is not felt.

On the other hand, a restricted apex presents a high current density, thus requiring an increased force (volts) to send the amperage through the apex. The higher the voltage or force, the more likely to reach the pain threshold.

We have all experienced this concept. Just think about the spark generated as your fingertip approaches a metal doorknob on a winter's day. Since the area struck by the spark is small, we feel the shock. However, if we were to grab the knob with the entire palm of our hand, the charge is not felt due to the greatly diminished current density even though there is an equivalent flow amperage through your hand.

A question arises in that if the voltage is insufficient to send a current through the apex how does it complete the circuit to turn on the EPT?

It is simply that the charge is sent through the entire tooth and exits through the entire root surface(a large surface area with a very low current density). This minimal force (volts) is insufficient to reach the thresholds of the sensory nerves but sufficient to activate the internal circuit in the pulp tester.

This concept of current density readily explains why deciduous teeth and newly erupted teeth with open apices may not respond to the electric pulp tester [11]. Even though the maximum output is reached, it also explains why teeth with multiple apices respond at higher ordinal readings.[2]

When the circuit is closed, the internal chip activates a program that incrementally increases the voltage till the unit maxes out at "80" or the circuit is broken. A void in the pulp chamber caused by necrosis of the pulp tissue in the chamber will prevent continuity of the circuit and the patient will not feel the charge. The

[2] Recall ordinal readings on an EPT is not equal to actual voltage. So, a reading of 30 on one tooth does not equate to a reading of 30 on another tooth… even on the same person.

resultant interpretation is that the pulp is necrotic. This is the prime reason EPTs should be considered a continuity meter and not a vitality meter.

Parenthetically, there may be vital (but diseased) tissue remaining further down the canal. Unless there is a clear indication (a periapical radiolucency or PARL) that the tooth is abscessed proceed with treatment as if there is still some remaining pulp capable of transmitting pain. Local anesthesia may be required to adequately instrument the canal comfortably since viable tissue may remain deep within the canal.

A caveat to this premise is that pus and even blood can act as electrolyte and a chamber filled with either can conduct the electric charge to remaining vital tissue juxtaposed to the apex thus mimicking a vital pulp.

Another concern is that the charge can be sent to an adjacent tooth via the proximal contacts. If this is suspected, the continuity may be interrupted by placing a mylar strip separating the contacts.

On the other hand, if a "small" part of the uninsulated probe touches a small area of the mucosa an intense shock may be delivered due to the small area of contact resulting in a high current density. *Supplemental information on Current Density is provided in the addendum.*

4.3 Helpful Hints in Use of the Electric Pulp Tester

(a) An often-overlooked concern is that the EPT probe tip has lost its coating or non-conductive protective sleeve as a result of repeated sterilization. If the uninsulated probe contacts soft tissue (i.e., cheek mucosa), current flow may short circuit and not pass through the pulp canal at a high enough voltage to activate the threshold potential.
(b) When re-testing, allow the EPT to reset to "0" before re-applying it to the tooth.
(c) Readings of 80 (maximum) *do not necessarily indicate* the pulp is non-vital. There may be vital tissue deep in the canal, but the circuit was not completed due to a void created by necrosis of the tissue in the pulp chamber or excess reparative dentin as increased the impedance so great that the voltage could not overcome it. An equally important reason for a failure to respond is an open apex resulting in a low current density.
(d) Failure of the EPT to turn on is due to a failure to complete the circuit. Make sure the patient grounds the wand with his fingers. If the unit does not turn on, it may be that the fingers are too dry, especially in construction workers or the elderly with dry skin. Moisten the fingers with some toothpaste. This will complete the circuit and the tester will turn on.
(e) Teeth with large restorations, extensive decay, or reparative dentin tend to have higher readings.
(f) Primary teeth and teeth with open apexes may fail to respond or give unreliable test results. This failure to respond is best explained by current density *(see discussion on Current Density).*
(g) Keep area isolated moisture (saliva) free... Air-dry the tooth. It is not sufficient to dry the tooth with gauze since moisture at the proximal contacts may conduct

the electric charge to adjacent teeth. Contact with soft tissue will invalidate readings by short-circuiting to adjacent tissues.

(h) If results from testing multi-rooted teeth are inconclusive test the buccal or lingual (palatal) surface of individual cusps. Partial pulp necrosis may prevent completion of the circuit from the contact area that is overlying the necrotic pulp. A fractured cusp may interrupt the flow of EC and result in no response at "80" even though the pulp may still be vital. A large restoration or caries can also block the flow of current to the pulp.

(i) It has been noted that teeth recently moved by orthodontic means or teeth suffering from recent trauma (within 72 h) may fail to respond to the pulp tester. These teeth should be considered vital when additional signs and symptoms of non-vitality are lacking. Periodic follow-up in 72 h is prudent, then again after 2 weeks, 2 months, and again at 6 months following trauma. Necrobiosis (partial pulp necrosis) may occur long after an initial incident.

(j) Patients with teeth that are extremely painful to touch (SAP) may be tested by contacting the tooth with the prob. tip and withdrawing it 1–2 mm retaining a strand of toothpaste to maintain a closed circuit. This way the patient will not confuse the pulpal pain with pressure exerted on sensitive PDL by the probe tip.

(k) Some toothpastes have been found to be unsatisfactory conductors of electric charges. Read the manufacturer's directions as to use of a conducting paste [12, 13].

4.3.1 Occlusal Analysis

Pain caused by trauma usually arises from the PDL. If trauma from occlusion is suspected, articulating paper may be used to identify premature contacts. Premature contacts may also be detected by placing the index finger half on the facial surface of the tooth and half on the alveolus, feeling for the impact (fremitus) as the teeth occlude or move under lateral excursions.

When using articulating paper to determine premature contacts, I have found the red-blue paper the most accurate when used in the following manner. Mark the questioned arch with red and the opposing arch with blue. Make sure to adequately dry the occlusal surfaces of upper and lower teeth with air and gauze prior to marking. Once adequate marks are observed, have the patient tap their teeth together in centric relation without any articulating paper in place so that the blue markings transfer to the red marking on the suspect teeth resulting in a purple color. This will indicate the premature contacts. Repeat the process having the patient mark interference areas with excursive movements.

4.3.2 Cracked Tooth

Cracked teeth are often a source of intense sharp pain upon biting, which may be difficult for the patient to localize if it does not involve the PDL. At one time, methylene blue dye was used to trace a suspected fracture. It was sealed in with a temporary restoration and reevaluated after several days allowing the dye to stain the fracture. This procedure has become obsolete with the availability of endodontic scopes and loops that have greatly improved visibility. However, scopes are not practical nor affordable for the general practitioner.

A simpler method of determining the presence of a fracture involves the use of the patients' biting force to create a painful response. Sharp pain may be elicited from a fractured tooth by challenging the cusps individually with an orangewood stick, an orthodontic band seater, or a small cotton ball placed in position so as to wedge the cusps apart. A device called the "Tooth Slooth®" directs occlusal forces to individual cusps making the fractured cusp readily identifiable. It overcomes some of the problems associated with the other testing methods by distributing forces to a well-defined cusp.

A minute fracture (especially one that is confined to enamel) may be suspected when the patient bites firmly without discomfort but experiences a sharp pain upon rapidly releasing the biting pressure. A larger fracture will likely respond as occlusal forces are applied either biting or releasing. When all else fails, yet a cracked tooth is still suspected, band the tooth, and send patient home. Note any change in symptoms over 2–4 days with band in place. A decrease of pain following banding may indicate a cracked tooth (this is rarely done in today's world.)

An important point to keep in mind is that any force applied occlusally will transmit to the apex and therefore any report of pain must differentiate sharp dentinal pain from apical periodontitis. Note, a cracked tooth (if vital) will elicit a dentinal (sharp) pain while the tooth with an apical periodontitis will elicit a sore aching type of pain. *Can you explain why this should be so?*

Visual evaluation of the crown, along with transillumination, should help to distinguish the cracked tooth from one with acute apical periodontitis. Be mindful, a non-vital cracked tooth will be painful if the crack extends to the PDL (see Chap. 3.)

Fremitus is another diagnostic aid helpful in determining the location of a fracture gingival, middle, or apical third. Place a finger on the buccal of the root and wiggle the crown buccal-lingually. Any crepitus (vibration) felt results from the separate parts of the fracture tooth rubbing together.

4.3.3 Dentinal Sensitivity (DS) or Test Cavity Preparation

Vitality may also be determined simply by scratching an area of exposed dentin with an explorer or directing a gentle air stream on exposed dentin. The quality of pain elicited should be sharp with minimal lingering effects. Intense pain is characteristic of dentinal hypersensitivity (DH) and suggests an allodynia. On the other hand, should spontaneous aching pain develop the pulp is likely undergoing an inflammatory process that could result in necrobiosis, eventually becoming completely necrotic necessitating RCT or extraction.

It is difficult to test teeth for vitality that are heavily restored or have full coverage. As a last resort the crown may be removed, or a test cavity can be prepared by drilling through the occlusal surface of the crown. The opening should be large enough to allow for proper placement of the EPT probe and conduction medium (not touching metal). Be sure to expose sufficient dentin to be tested with the EPT probe. Often dentinal sensitivity or a "foul odor" emanating from the preparation will preclude the need of having to use the EPT and restoration is best determined by removal of the entire restoration to evaluate prognosis. The test cavity should be prepared in the location endodontic access dictates. This will prevent unnecessary damage to the remaining tooth structure if endodontic treatment is indicated and the underlying tooth structure is intact and not carious. The access can then be sealed with a non-conductive restorative material to prevent a galvanic reaction.

4.3.4 Selective Local Anesthesia

You will encounter cases in which all signs and symptoms point to one offending tooth and the patient points to another tooth, sometimes in the opposing arch (referred pain). Differentiating between two suspect teeth is often best accomplished by selective local anesthesia. In cases where the same nerve enervates the suspected teeth local infiltration or PDL injection may be helpful in localizing the offending tooth, but its reliability has been questioned [14]. Sub-periosteal injections may offer some discrimination [15]. The value of selective local anesthesia is often appreciated when pain is referred from one arch to the ipsilateral arch.

Very often a patient will identify retained roots of a lower molar as the offending tooth when the chief complaint reported was "sensitive to cold." Since the retained roots are most likely non-vital, the patient may be experiencing referred pain from a vital but carious maxillary molar with pulpitis. The status of the pulp would depend on the onset of the pain. Selective anesthesia may convince the patient that the retained roots are not the source of pain and readily accepts your professional judgment to treat the opposing tooth in spite of having been convinced it was the broken-down molar.

4.3.5 Radiographic Findings

The final step in the data collection process is a radiographic survey. In an effort to expedite the diagnostic work-up, there is a tendency to order the imaging before the visual exam. In so doing, it is possible to expose a radiographic film that is of little value. This is especially true for toothaches characterized by referred pain. Ideally a radiograph should be ordered to confirm a tentative diagnosis after an initial clinical evaluation has been performed. Doing so allows the proper selection of the type of radiograph, as well as area and angulation. Following a visual examination, the radiograph may confirm your diagnosis, or it can be of value tracing a sinus tract with a gutta percha cone. Although the radiograph is a valuable tool, it should not be the sole test to rely on for a final diagnosis.

When having to treat a new patient without a "treatment plan" it is helpful to have a full mouth scan (panoramic view) so as to determine the best course of action. This allows taking the overall oral condition of the mouth and formulating a treatment goal before initiating treatment of a specific tooth.

References

1. Brännström M, Astroem A. A study on the mechanism of pain elicited from the dentin. J Dent Res. 1964;43:619–25. https://doi.org/10.1177/00220345640430041601. PMID:14183350.
2. Brännström M. The hydrodynamic theory of dentinal pain: sensation in preparations, caries, and the dentinal crack syndrome. J Endod. 1986;12(10):453–7. https://doi.org/10.1016/S0099-2399(86)80198-4. PMID: 3465849.
3. Van Hassel HJ. Physiology of human dental pulp. Oral Surg Oral Med Oral Pathol. 1971;32(1):126–34. https://doi.org/10.1016/0030-4220(71)90258-1. PMID: 5281545.
4. Minoux M, Serfaty R. Vital tooth bleaching: biologic adverse effects-a review. Quintessence Int. 2008;39(8):645–59. PMID: 19107251.
5. Wang C-W, Wang K-L, Ho K-H, Hsieh S-C, Chang H-M. Dental pulp response to orthodontic tooth movement. Taiwanese J Orthod. 2017;29(4):2. https://doi.org/10.30036/TJO.201712_29(4).0002.
6. Seltzer S, Bender IB, Ziontz M. The dynamics of pulp inflammation: correlations between diagnostic data and actual histologic findings in the pulp. Oral Surg Oral Med Oral Pathol. 1963;16:846–71. https://doi.org/10.1016/0030-4220(63)90323-2. PMID: 13987830.
7. Weisleder R, Yamauchi S, Caplan DJ, Trope M, Teixeira FB. The validity of pulp testing: a clinical study. J Am Dent Assoc. 2009;140(8):1013–7. https://doi.org/10.14219/jada.archive.2009.0312. PMID: 19654254.
8. Jespersen JJ, Hellstein J, Williamson A, Johnson WT, Qian F. Evaluation of dental pulp sensibility tests in a clinical setting. J Endod. 2014;40(3):351–4. https://doi.org/10.1016/j.joen.2013.11.009. Epub 2013 Dec 15. PMID: 24565651.
9. Lado EA, Richmond AF, Marks RG. Reliability and validity of a digital pulp tester as a test standard for measuring sensory perception. J Endod. 1988;14(7):352–6. https://doi.org/10.1016/S0099-2399(88)80197-3. PMID: 3251997.
10. <https://en.wikipedia.org/wiki/Electrical_resistivity_and_conductivity>.
11. https://physics.info/electric-current/.
12. Instruction pamphlet for digital EPT (Point 3 Frequently asked questions about the Vitality Scanner) provided by SybronEndo, 1332 South Lone Hill Ave, Glendora, CA 91740.
13. Mickel AK, Kimberly AD, et al. Electric pulp tester conductance through various Interface media. JOE. 2006;32(12):1179–80. https://doi.org/10.1016/j.joen.2006.06.009.
14. Wong JK. Adjuncts to local anesthesiza: separating fact from fiction. J Can Dent Assoc. 2001;67(7):391–7. PMID: 1148097.
15. Esnaashari E, Mirzaei S, Moshari A, Razavi P. Onset of action and duration of efficacy of inferior alveolar nerve block versus single lingual subperi-osteal injection of 4% articaine in mandibular second molars: a randomized clinical trial. J Res Dent Maxillofac Sci. 2022;7(3):119–24. https://doi.org/10.52547/jrdms.7.3.119.

Periodontal Disease 5

5.1 Introduction

The periodontium is the attachment apparatus of the dental complex that is comprised of gingiva, cementum, periodontal ligaments, (PDL), and alveolar bone. The principal function includes supporting and protecting teeth and their pulps from injury caused by mechanical forces. In effect, the PDL not only holds the teeth in place but acts as a shock absorber of forces applied to the tooth. It is amply supplied with sensory nerves as well as proprioceptive fibers allowing for localization of pain reported by the patient. Recall proprioceptive fibers are not found in the dental pulp. C-fibers provide the predominant pain afferent nerves to the periodontium and a spontaneous dull-aching pain predominates.

When injured, a sharp shooting "**neuropathic pain**" may be elicited from nerve fibers located in the periodontium. This pain mimics pain associated with a-∂ and C-nerve fibers and should not be interpreted as pulp pain. Neuropathic pain may be caused by multiple diseases, such as diabetes or injury resulting in damage to the nerves. It can present as abnormal sensations such as numbness or tingling to a sharp stinging or a burning sensation. It can be continuous and/or episodic spontaneous and/or elicited. Common qualities include burning or coldness, "pins and needles" sensations, numbness, and itching often behaving as an "Allodynia" (a painful response to a normally non-painful stimulus). The difference is that neuropathic pain presents a variety of symptoms as compared to the predictable pain propagated from a-∂ and C-fibers.

5.1.1 Normal Periodontium

Healthy gingiva is pink, non-tender, does not bleed during normal function and is firmly attached to the tooth. Any swelling, redness, tenderness, foul odor, metallic taste, or unprovoked bleeding is a common finding in periodontal disease. Most

E. Lado, R. Caudle, *Pathway to Diagnosis and Management of Toothaches*,
https://doi.org/10.1007/978-3-031-75262-9_5

diseases affecting the periodontium are inflammatory and may arise from several factors including mechanical/physical trauma, food impaction, pathogens, immune diseases, nutritional deficiencies, side effects of some medications, and overall poor oral hygiene.

The periodontium can harbor disease at any level of the alveolus including the operculum (tissue overlying the occlusal portion of the crown). The operculum over third molars is often traumatized by the opposing tooth and/or infected by bacteria trapped in the underlying pseudo-pocket. Affected root levels may be divided into 3 segments based on location: "Marginal" (coronal area to the gingival attachment), "Radicular" (area along the side of the root where periodontal ligaments attach), and "Apical" (area where blood vessels and nerve fibers enter and exit the pulp chamber of the tooth).

5.1.2 Inflamed Periodontium

See Table 5.1.

The following elaborates on the above table.

1. ***Marginal Periodontitis***: can arise for a number of reasons most all will ultimately manifest as an infection. Visual inspection, periodontal probing, and history of the chief complaint are usually sufficient to arrive at a diagnosis. Patients usually complain of an aching sensation with swollen and tender gums that bleed easily. The typical pain associated with a pulp problem is not present unless there is exposed dentin due to gingival recession, or abrasion/abfraction exposing dentinal tubules. When viable dentinal tubules are exposed to tactile, thermal, or chemical (acidic) challenges, a sharp pain may prevail.
   (a) *Food Impaction*: (a common complaint) usually recures in specific locations. Patients will complain of a nagging *aching* pain especially after eating if food wedges between teeth or is packed into a periodontal pocket. It will be tender to probing, may become swollen, and likely to bleed easily. Localized marginal swelling is characteristic of a marginal (gingival) abscess.
   (b) *Gingivitis*: Generalized inflammatory reaction to accumulations of bacteria and plaque. Gingiva becomes tender and bleeds easily. The most common

Table 5.1 Type of Inflamed Periodontium by Location

Marginal Periodontitis	*Radicular Periodontitis*	*Apical Periodontitis*
Food impaction, plaque and calculus accumulation	*Pocket formation, with bone loss*	*Occlusal trauma, pulp inflammation*
Gingivitis, Pericoronitis, Operculitis	*Lateral periodontal abscess Fractured root*	*Pulp necrosis, Necrobiosis Apical abscess*
Immune response ANUG	*Developmental pathologic abnormality*	*Inflammation of surrounding tissues (sinusitis)*

cause is inadequate home care and diet. Treatment should include professional debridement, proper home care, and diet counseling. An Rx for chlorhexidine gluconate 0.12% may help speed the resolution of the inflammatory process.

(c) *Pericoronitis/Operculitis*: is a swelling commonly seen around erupting third molars. Patients usually complain of a continuous aching pain that is exacerbated by a "sharp" pain upon biting and swallowing. The patient is likely to have an opposing tooth traumatizing the swollen area. Extraction of the opposing tooth should be considered as a temporary measure to alleviate pain. The pocket may require debridement and irrigation with chlorhexidine gluconate 0.12%. They should also be given an Rx for chlorhexidine gluconate 0.12% and instructed to rinse BID after eating and brushing along with an appropriate antibiotic. Arrangements should be made to remove the tooth as soon as is practical. Preferably prior to completion of the course of antibiotic. Since fascial space infections are a risk with third molar infections, definitive treatment should be provided as soon as possible. NOTE: Be sure to check for a space infection.

(d) *Immune Response*: An immune response could result from stress, a vitamin C deficiency, pregnancy gingivitis, ANUG, leukemia, to a hodgepodge of oral diseases. The patient should be referred to their PCP for further evaluation if the condition fails to respond to normal dental treatment including gentle debridement, diet and stress counseling, Vit C and B complex supplements, topical analgesics, frequent saline rinses especially following eating, chlorhexidine gluconate 0.12% rinses twice a day. Schedule for a thorough cleaning once condition begins to resolve. Consider Rx for antibiotic if systemic symptoms of infection are present or patient has diabetes/uncontrolled or other immune deficiencies.

2. ***Radicular Periodontitis***: (Refer to Fig. 5.1 Schematic section) Inflammation along the lateral border of the root.

   (a) *Periodontal Pockets W/Bone Loss*: Pockets greater than 3 mm present an ongoing problem for the patient. Even with flossing, food, and bacteria harbor in the depth of the pocket. Eventually, inflammation will result in increased pocket depth and loss of bone supporting the tooth. A water irrigating device or a proxy-brush may be helpful if removing food trapped in an embrasure but are not a substitute for flossing and routine prophylaxis. Meticulous care may retard the process, but eventually periodontal surgery to reduce the pocket depth or extraction may be necessary.

   (b) *Lateral Periodontal Abscess*: can be an elusive diagnosis. The presence of a sinus tract and swelling can mimic a draining apical abscess (chronic apical abscess). This abscess is often caused by a tooth fracture extending to the PDL attachment. Another common cause of such an abscess is a nidus of calculus allowed to remain following a deep periodontal scaling where reattachment of the periodontium occurs occlusal to trapped debris.

   It can also occur from a lateral accessory canal if the pulp is necrosing. Treatment is causal dependent, often requiring drainage. Diagnosis is

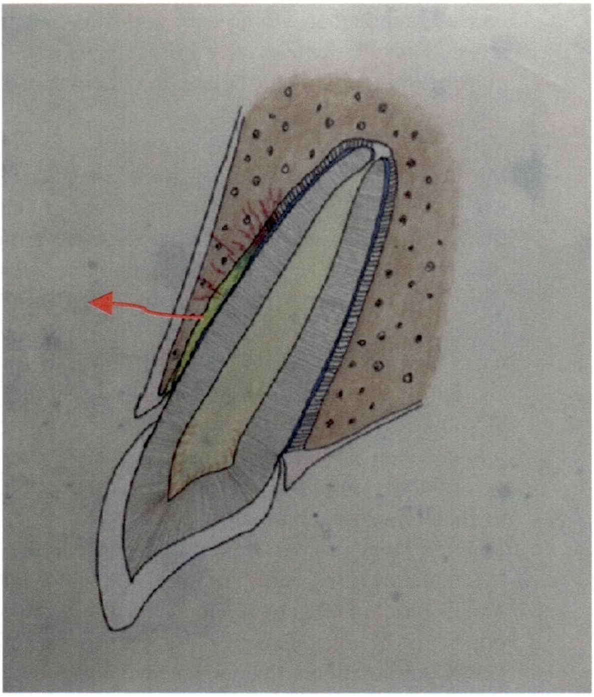

Fig. 5.1 Lateral Periodontal Abscess*. * OLD TERMINOLOGY

facilitated by tracing a sinus tract with a gutta percha cone if possible and confirming the terminal path with radiographic imaging. Restorability will be a major consideration as to the preferred treatment.

(c) *Developmental/Pathologic Abnormalities*: such as cysts arising from tooth development can also mimic a lateral periodontal abscess radiographically and be asymptomatic unless they become infected.

3. ***Apical Periodontitis***: is an inflammatory response to trauma or infection found at the apex of the tooth. It is characterized by pain upon biting and sensitivity to percussion. Basically, it is an aching pain originating from C-fibers located within the PDL.

   (a) *Occlusal Trauma*: (Refer to Fig. 5.2 Schematic section) may occur from clenching/bruxing. A restoration in hyper occlusion, an ill-fitting prothesis, a functional change in occlusion, orthodontics, etc., can all cause tactile allodynia or possibly bruising of the periodontium initiating the production of PgE_2. This pain mediator lowers the pain threshold of the nerves supplying the pulp and can even cause them to become sensitive to thermal stimulation. This is not due to an infection and does not warrant antibiotics. Occlusal adjustment or a bruxing appliance along with an anti-inflammatory analgesic will usually resolve the problems. Depending on the severity of the trauma and production of PgE_2, the surrounding tissues may become tender to palpation.

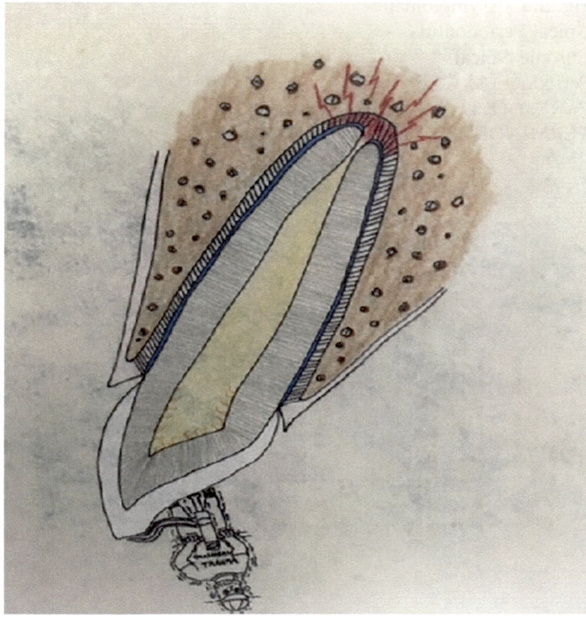

Fig. 5.2 Symptomatic apical periodontitis (SAP) Acute apical periodontitis*. * OLD TERMINOLOGY

(b) *Inflammation of Surrounding Tissues*: A common cause of apical periodontitis is inflammation arising from the sinuses. Prostaglandins (PgE_2) produced in conjunction with an inflamed sinus will lower the pain thresholds of nerves supplying the proximal dentition and periodontium. It is essential to rule-out sinusitis prior to condemning a suspect tooth to extraction or RCT. Usually, the patient is aware of a sinus condition, but palpation of the maxillary and frontal sinuses may be revealing.

(c) *Sterile Pulpitis/Necrosis*: can lead to asymptomatic apical periodontitis (AAP or symptomatic apical periodontitis (SAP). Sterile pulpitis and necroses can arise from a failed pulp cap, a traumatic blow severing the blood supply to the pulp or improper etching and/or curing of a composite restoration. This may be evidenced by internal resorption when the odontoclasts, from the pulp, attack the dentin that has been denatured by application of caustic chemicals.

(d) *Asymptomatic Apical Periodontitis*: (Refer to Fig. 5.3 Schematic section) (AAP) Previously referred to as chronic apical periodontitis (CAP) results from a dying pulp leaving the apex non-biocompatible. AAE defines it as an "inflammation and destruction of the apical periodontium that is of pulpal origin" but does not explain the cause or progression of the process that gave rise to the destruction of bone at the apex. "It appears as an apical radiolucency and does not present clinical symptoms (no pain on percussion or palpation)." This definition is wanting since there is no explanation as to the progression of the condition from when it first exited the apex and entered

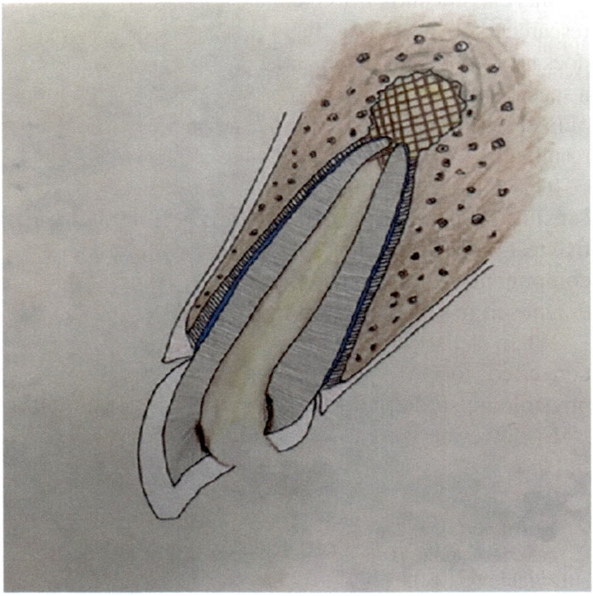

Fig. 5.3 Asymptomatic Apical Periodontitis. Chronic Apical Periodontitis* CAP* PARL. * OLD TERMINOLOGY

the PDL. My assumption is that it initially did present some minimal clinical symptoms and was radiographically imperceptible, but as time went on a periapical radiolucency (PARL) appeared that increased in size significantly without causing any notable discomfort.

I find it hard to accept an inflamed/dying pulp did not produce sufficient amounts of prostaglandins to lower the pain thresholds of the afferent neurons in the PDL to cause pain with one major exception. That is the pulp died quietly (apoptosis), i.e., trauma severing the blood supply, failed pulp cap, caustic restoration, acid etching, frictional heating of the pulp, or any other means of a sterile necrosis. In which case the levels of PgE_2 could have been low enough so as not to provoke pain other than the initial pain associated with the cause. Since pathogenic activity was nil, cell lysis and bone resorption occurred slowly thereby the amount of PgE_2 concentrated in the area was minimal, and the threshold for perceiving pain was sufficiently lowered so as not to cause discomfort. This condition can exist for years without the patient being aware and is often discovered upon radiographic examination where a large PARL may be seen.

(e) *Symptomatic Apical Periodontitis*: (Refer to Fig. 5.2 Schematic section) AAE defines SAP as “inflammation, usually of the apical periodontium, producing clinical symptoms involving a painful response to biting and/or percussion or palpation. This may or may not be accompanied by radiographic changes (i.e., depending upon the stage of the disease, there may be normal width of the periodontal ligament or there may be a periapical radiolucency). Severe pain to percussion and/or palpation is highly indicative of a degenerating pulp and root canal treatment is needed."

I find this definition extremely limiting since pain upon percussion can have multiple causes including occlusal trauma, bruxism, or even inflammation of nearby structures such as an inflamed sinus. It is characterized by sensitivity to occlusal forces (biting) and percussion but *not to palpation*. Failure to improve, following addressing a suspected non-odontogenic etiology, suggests the progression of pulpal involvement If the apical area becomes sensitive to palpation the level of PgE_2 has increased significantly and is highly suggestive of development of an apical abscess.

(f) *Acute Apical Abscess*: (Refer to Figs. 5.4 and 5.5 Schematic section) occurs when bacteria enter the apical area of the tooth socket and kill the surrounding cells producing much higher levels of PgE_2 this lowers the pain threshold of the associated C-fibers resulting in a severe continuous aching pain. The area will not only remain sensitive to percussion but will also become sensitive to touch (palpation). This sensitivity to palpation results from a dramatic increase of PgE_2 and swelling results due to an accumulation of edematous fluid (cellulitis). At this time, an abscess exists in bone with a generalized inflammatory response occurring in the surrounding tissue. As the abscess erodes through the cortical bone and periosteum pus coalesces presenting a fluctuant swelling. A diagnosis of an abscess may be made even when swelling is not present based on the presence of pain to touch and palpation of the apical area. The pain associated with an apical abscess takes on an aching quality associated with C-fibers as opposed to a sharp shooting pain associated with a-∂ fibers. In fact, the pain associated with an apical abscess is usually less intensive than that associated with pulpitis in that the contents of a pulpal abscess are confined within a ridged structure and cannot accommodate for the edema. A cold compress is unlikely to provoke pain but can provide some relief by reducing swelling (edema).

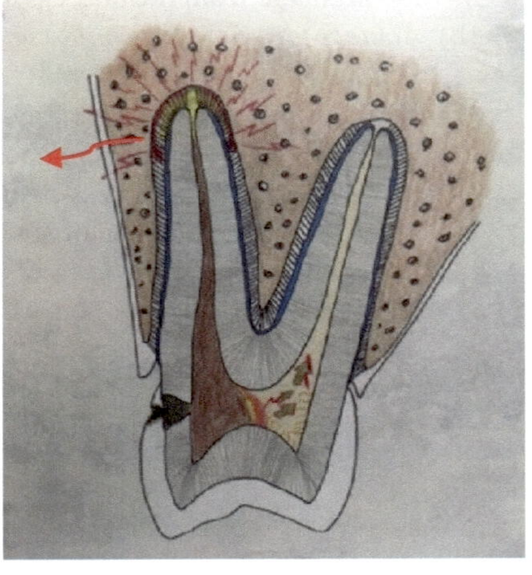

Fig. 5.4 SIP/Acute Apical Abscess. IP/AAA*. * OLD TERMINOLOGY

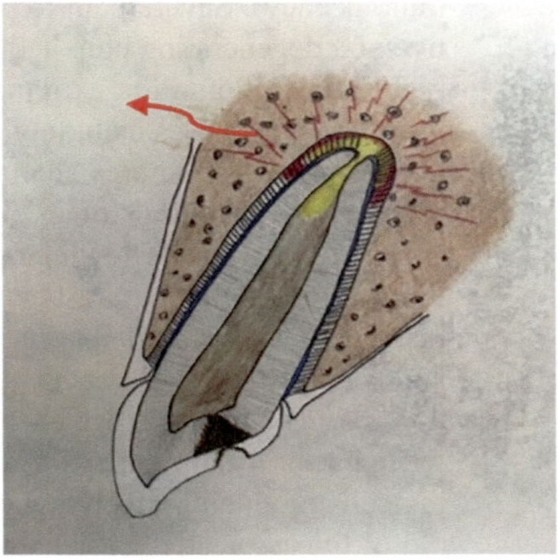

Fig. 5.5 Necrotic pulp/ Acute Apical Abscess. NP/ AAA*. * OLD TERMINOLOGY

Prior to the occurrence of the abscess in soft tissue, cellulitis may occur resulting in a firm diffuse swelling as well as tenderness to the surrounding area due to the accumulation of fluid in the area. (edema). A radiographic lucency may not be evident if the root apex is fenestrated but may have a history of swelling suggesting an abscess. Also, it usually takes several days for sufficient bone to be destroyed by an abscess (PARL) to show on a radiographic image.

(g) *Chronic Apical Abscess*: (Refer to Fig. 5.6 Schematic section (CAA) is a term that is presently used by AAE to signify the presence of a sinus tract draining pus from an apical lesion. In the former terminology it was called chronic suppurative apical periodontitis (CSAP). Little pain accompanies this condition since the sinus tract provides an egress for pus and other inflammatory exudates. An open pulp canal can also provide drainage as does the sinus tract and similar symptoms exist. The danger comes should the patient decide to place an OTC dental stopping in the cavity (blocking the drainage from the abscess and significant pain will likely occur).

(h) *Acute Flare-up of Asymptomatic Apical Periodontitis*: (Refer to Fig. 5.7 Schematic section (AF-AAP) occurs when bacteria find their way to the affected area of an AAP (previously called a chronic apical periodontitis). They may enter through an open necrotic pulp canal or even via the circulatory system by the process of anachoresis. If bacteria overwhelm the body's defenses an acute apical abscess (AAA) develops. The term "Phoenix Abscess" was previously used to denote an acute flare-up of an asymptomatic (Chronic) apical lesion. Histologically, it is no different from an acute apical abscess and presents the same clinical symptoms. The major difference is that the radiolucent area of a Phoenix abscess can be significantly larger than the early onset of an acute apical abscess. Phoenix abscess has also been used to connote a failed root canal treatment.

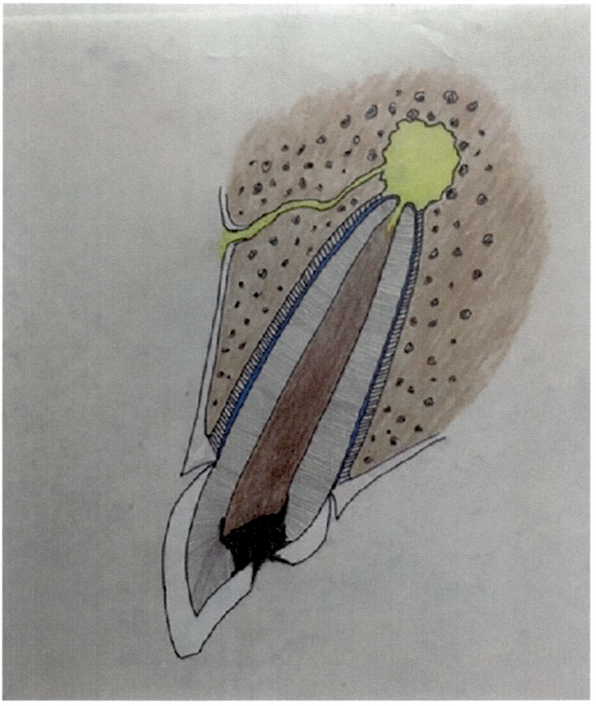

Fig. 5.6 Chronic Apical Abscess (note sinus tract. Chronic Suppurative Apical Periodontitis*). PARL. * OLD TERMINOLOGY

NOTE: *Judgment to prescribe antibiotics depends heavily on severity of the abscess, systemic involvement, fever, involvement of fascial spaces, comorbidities (immunity, diabetes, medications, recent surgeries, and the like). Use of antibiotics for pulpal involvement without periodontal involvement is not justified. Antibiotics do not enter a necrosing pulp; however, if there is an indication that the periodontium is involved amoxicillin or Augmentin is recommended or clindamycin if the patient is allergic to penicillin-based antibiotics*

5.1.3 Endo-Perio Diagnosis

Most toothaches present as a combination pulp and periodontal pathology. We have discussed pulp and periodontal pathosis separately, but it is time to begin considering the tooth and alveolus as a unit.

Once the PDL is involved, a proper diagnosis of tooth pain demands one that reflects the health of each component of the involved odontogenic complex. Thus, the diagnosis should appear with the status of the pulp first and the periodontium following, i.e., symptomatic irreversible pulpitis/acute apical abscess.

At first glance, this diagnosis appears reasonable; however, if this were a single rooted tooth, there would not be a blood supply keeping the pulp alive so rather than

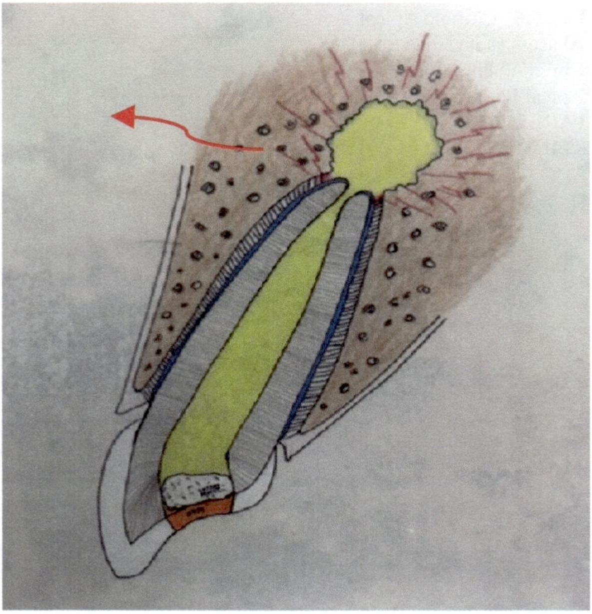

Fig. 5.7 Asymptomatic PARL becomes symptomatic. Phoenix Abscess*??? Necrotic pulp/AAA. Periapical radiolucency PARL. History of long standing PARL. * *OLD TERMINOLOGY*

call it irreversible, we have to refer to it as necrotic. On the other hand, if this was a multirooted tooth, it could be perfectly reasonable. An abscess may form on one root while the remaining roots could supply nutrients to the remaining inflamed pulp. The point being the diagnosis should reflect the most severe condition on which treatment will be based.

Another consideration after having diagnosed a diseased tooth is to evaluate how it needs to be restored and how it would fit into the overall treatment plan before discussing treatment options for a single tooth with the patient. The overall treatment plan and cost should be accepted by the patient before recommending a costly procedure with which the patient will not comply.

Endo-Perio. Diagnosis results in loss of periodontal support due to pulp necroses passing through an accessory canal to the PDL. By treating and resolving the pulpal infection, the destroyed bone may reform. On the other hand, a Perio-Endo lesion has a guarded prognosis and is dependent on the remaining bone following periodontal treatment. In this case, the pulp becomes infected through an accessory canal exposed by the loss of bone. The RCT will not promote new bone to regenerate, so the outcome is not only dependent on a successful RCT but also on the remaining bone support. In rare cases where the accessory canal is close to the marginal gingival attachment level, the prognosis will be more favorable. This later situation may be found in molars where the accessory canal terminates in the furcation.

6 Addendum

6.1 Systematic Approach

A well-planned approach to the diagnosis of toothaches prevents wasting time conducting unnecessary tests and putting patients through additional unnecessary discomfort. The following schema is offered to facilitate your approach to diagnose toothaches.

1. *Once the necessary demographics have been collected the patient should express their Chief Complaint (CC) by responding to the question (What brought you in today?) This answer should be unambiguous as to the precise problem… not "I have a toothache", rather something along the lines of "I have had a toothache on the lower right side for a couple of days and it is keeping me up at night." If they do not volunteer the added information take the time to ask appropriate follow-up questions. This should give you an idea as to how to proceed with your evaluation.*
2. *Once the CC is established it is critical to proceed with a thorough review of the medical history including recent visits to their PCP, a review of medications prescribed, as well as any/all OTC remedies they have recently taken, including analgesics, vitamins, herbals, and antacids. It is also important to ask if they have attempted to relieve their pain with OTC toothache remedies since they can interfere with the findings from diagnostic tests. A question that should not be avoided for fear of offending a patient is the use of recreational drugs especially cocaine that can be used to quell dental pain.*
3. *At this point, vitals may be recorded if they have yet to be done.*
4. *Proceed with the external examination by noting any changes in consistency or color of the skin and facial asymmetry. Palpate the head and neck including the maxillary and frontal sinuses as well as the temporal area and TMJ noting any*

E. Lado, R. Caudle, *Pathway to Diagnosis and Management of Toothaches*,
https://doi.org/10.1007/978-3-031-75262-9_6

swelling, tenderness, or crepitus. Palpation of the submaxillary, cervical, and postauricular nodes is warranted especially on the ipsilateral side as the chief complaint.

5. *The intraoral exam should begin with examination of the tongue (especially the posterior and lateral borders), floor of mouth, palate cheek and vestibular areas of the mucosa. The condition of the gingiva and vestibular area can be reveling. Note any swelling, sinus tracts, ulcerations, traumatic injuries, and chemical burns. Sloughing white mucosa is often evidence of an aspirin burn caused by the patient attempting relief by placing an aspirin on the affected area. While an ulcerated lateral border of the tongue or cheek may have been caused by a broken crown with sharp protrusions.*
6. *Other OTC remedies, such as eugenol, can also cause sloughing of mucosa* [1]·
7. *Several distressing pathologic conditions present on the oral mucosa. Any abnormal finding should be investigated.*
8. *Once you have determined that treatment will require an irreversible procedure (extraction, RCT,* etc.*) there is a tendency to initiate a discussion reviewing alternative treatments with the patient. No matter how sure you are of the diagnosis… you should refrain from discussing possible treatment options until the condition of the entire dentition has been established and formulation of a treatment plan is in process.*
9. *It is now time to proceed with a radiographic study (panoramic view). This will allow an inclusive evaluation of the importance of retaining a tooth* vs. *extraction. It also calls attention to pathologic findings that could have a major effect on treatments.*
10. *Once this information is accumulated and processed, you may now proceed with appropriate diagnostic testing. For instance, thermal testing of a partially impacted third molar designated for extraction would be inappropriate and put the patient through unnecessary discomfort.*
11. *Once you have a working diagnosis you may begin exploring treatment alternatives.*

6.2 Emergency Department Visits

When treating an emergency toothache, it is important to pinpoint the precise cause of the CC so that appropriate treatment may be rendered. Unfortunately, the oral condition of many patients seeking treatment at the Emergency Department (ED) is poor and the diagnosis is often obscured among a myriad of dental problems.

Most EDs are ill prepared to diagnose or manage toothaches. Narcotic analgesics and antibiotics are often the "go-to" remedy regardless of the diagnosis. At times the antibiotic scripted is not the best choice for the problem [2]. Understandably the trend to prescribing antibiotic is often warranted in warding off the spread of infection into fascial spaces or systemically but not every toothache presents such a problem and at times the diagnosis does not warrant antibiotics or strong analgesics.

Many patients that were seen in the ED wait to seek definitive dental care until after completing a course of prescribed medication and the pain returns. It is important to advise the patient to arrange for appropriate care as soon as possible and not wait till after they have completed the prescription, and the problem returns.

An appreciation of the causes of oral pain will help direct the ED provider toward appropriate care and prevent unnecessary medication. Sometimes the source of severe tooth pain is from the dental pulp or dentin (dentinal sensitivity) in which case an antibiotic is useless. Narcotic analgesics may block pain but a simple application of a topical anesthetic (benzocaine) or oil of clove (eugenol) may be equally effective without the risks associated with the use of narcotics and/or antibiotics. Inflamed gingiva may be best treated with a 0.12% chlorhexidine gluconate rinse BID until the patient can be evaluated and treated by their dentist.

If the pain is simply associated with a fractured tooth cutting, the tongue palliative treatment may simply be to place some soft wax over the dentin to protect the tongue from ulceration or isolating tooth structure from thermal and caustic irritants till the patient can see their dentist.

Simply put, a better understanding of the cause of "toothaches" leads to appropriate and effective management.

6.3 Pain Thresholds

In the first section (Chap. 1. "Tooth Pain"), you may have noticed the level of pain is rated by three intensities. The levels may be perceived in terms of thresholds.

Mild: Threshold of Sensation, "It annoying but I can function normally".

Moderate: Threshold of Pain "It hurts, but can be controlled with analgesics".

Severe: Threshold of Tolerance "It hurts so much I can't take it anymore."

Most published research uses a 0-10 sliding scale with zero interpreted as no pain and 10 to be the most intense pain imaginable. When doing a research study involving a significant number of volunteers, this makes for a reasonable and valid approach. Everyone's reaction to pain is unique and by using the expanded scale a valid conclusion is more likely to be derived by analyzing and combining data gathered from many subjects. In reality, the 1-10 scale is reduced to three levels as listed above.

When dealing with a single patient and not knowing one's tolerance for pain, the three levels provide ample information to make a reasonable clinical judgment. When I (EL) am able to make a distinction between a "4" or "7" reported by the patient, I will consider rethinking the 3 levels of intensity used to make a judgment on which my diagnosis and treatment will be based. Till then, my diagnoses will be heavily influenced by the characteristics and onset of pain and the intensity determining the urgency of treatment and/or the need for a stronger analgesic. Recall severe pain interferes with function, i.e., limited opening/difficulty swallowing/breathing, all requiring immediate attention. Any patient presenting with swelling, bleeding, systemic malaise, and fever requires evaluation STAT.

6.4 Control Teeth

Another grouse has to do with use of a "control tooth" when performing an EPT, thermal, and percussion test. Electric pulp test data from repeated tests over several days on the same subjects and teeth resulted in a wide variation of the ordinal readings for sensory and tolerance thresholds [3]. There are several reasons for inconsistent readings including amount of electrolyte used, the presence of secondary or reparative dentin, restorations, and undermining decay, dryness of the enamel, *size of the apex opening, (current density)* as well as operator technique and patient communication to mention a few, can all affect the EPT reading. Therefore, there is little reason to first test a contralateral tooth that is presumed healthy. In fact, testing a normal tooth first will only serve to alert the patient to the unpleasant sensation they are about to experience magnified by the pain they are already experiencing. To avoid the unwelcome discomfort the patient may react prematurely leading to a false positive reading on the suspected tooth. This concept also applies to thermal and percussion tests.

It is presumptuous to think a true "control" tooth can be selected simply by visual examination or selecting the contralateral equivalent as the target tooth. Equally presumptuous is to think that the target tooth will elicit similar responses to testing if it does not have pulpal or periodontal involved.

Recall, a number of conditions can affect a response to the various methods of testing. Parafunctional habits, sinus involvement, bruxism/clenching, bleaching, OTC toothache remedies, analgesics, anxiety, intense pain keeping the patient up with little or no sleep, restorations, acid etching, cracked tooth, allodynia, tarter control dentifrices, dietary habits/citrus acids, micro fractures in enamel (resulting in an allodynia), previous pulp capping, just to mention a few.

It is for this reason testing 4-5 neighboring teeth will help establish a patients' baseline reaction to a given stimulus and provide a better comparison of the test results obtained from the suspect offender.

All pertinent data should fit together like pieces of a puzzle. If something does not fit, make attempt to explain why, please do not attribute the baffling problem to the adage "It's all in her head." The patient may be right!

6.5 Non-Prescription Remedies

Some OTC "Toothache" remedies may be caustic to the gingiva and most provide directions for their proper use. Warn patients about placing aspirin-based powders (Goody Powder®) on the surrounding gingiva causing an acid burn of the surrounding soft tissue. According to label instructions, this product should be mixed with water and swallowed.

Some OTC remedies (Orabase®) are specifically intended to be placed on mucosal lesions such as aphthous ulcers. Irritated and inflamed gingiva may be managed with a.0.12% chlorhexidine gluconate BID and benzocaine lozenges or a maalox/

benadryl (see page 67) mouth rinse for oral ulcerations will help till the dentist can evaluate the cause of the inflammation and provide appropriate treatment.

If the problem is an acute ulcerative necrotizing gingivitis (ANUG) brought on by stress, high Vit C and B complex may also be appropriate along with stress reduction, proper nutrition, and rest. Antibiotics may be appropriate if the patient presents with fever and/or other systemic symptoms but is not the primary treatment of choice. The causative factors must be addressed.

Sore teeth upon mastication (Bruxing) may be temporarily relieved with the use of an inexpensive sports mouth guard. It is important to rule out sinus inflammation as the cause of tooth pain as well as referred pain from an opposing arch.

Food trapped in a deep periodontal pocket may result in a radicular periodontal abscess. Often attempts to remove food with dental floss succeed in driving the bolus deeper into the pocket. Trapped food may be best removed with an interdental brush. Should this be a recurring problem the patient may consult with their dentist about the use a water irrigation device (Waterpic®) being sure to direct the force of the spray perpendicular to the long axis of the tooth thus preventing driving the bolus of food deeper into the pocket.

There are a number of OTC remedies available to the patient. A better awareness of their use could help the patient manage their complaint till definitive measures can be taken.

I feel it is important to mention home care following treatment especially when it comes to surgery. It has been my experience that patients are instructed in managing their recovery period orally with a printout of the salient points. They are always asked. (Do you have any questions?) And invariably the response is "NO" …. (Thinking) just let me out of here! I am beat.)

I highly recommend a follow-up call and confirm the patient is doing "Okay."

While providing post-op instructions, discuss the need for analgesics and keeping their head elevated. Emphasize the importance of nutrition and if needed recommend a nutritional supplement available at any pharmacy or food store. You may also want to emphasize avoiding herbals that may interfere with clotting. Encourage your patient to do an internet search for side effects of any herbal they are taking especially ST. John's Wort [4]. This link may be of help.

6.6 Post-Op Care

Should post-op bleeding occur suggest activating a regular tea bag (NOT GREEN OR DECAFFEINATED) by placing it in hot water for a minute then wrapping it in gauze after expressing out the water. Place the wrapped tea bag over the extraction site with adequate pressure to stop bleeding. Maintain it in place for 30 minutes. Swallow (saliva/blood and solution expressed from tea bag while biting on it to control bleeding) as you would normally swallow your saliva. This should control bleeding. If it does not, a visit to the ED is appropriate.

A cold compress for the first few hours following extraction may help to keep swelling to a minimum. Should the patient develop difficulty swallowing or breathing, a visit to the ED as soon as possible is warranted.

As with any trauma, discomfort is expected. Warm rinses the day after oral surgery is often suggested. A saline solution was shown to be as effective as 0.12% chlorhexidine gluconate [5]. However, there is some question as to the effectiveness of copious irrigation immediately post-extraction. The study demonstrated that post-extraction socket bleeding is very important for the proper uncomplicated socket healing. If it is not washed away with irrigation solution at the end of extraction, the normal blood clot has a higher likelihood to form, and therefore, can potentially lead to an uncomplicated socket healing without development of alveolar osteitis [6].

6.7 Brännström's Hydrodynamic Theory of Dentin Hydrodynamics

A study by Martin Brännström on dentin sensitivity is a very interesting read. At the time, there were several hypotheses to explain dental sensitivity, but none were satisfactory. Dr. Brännström's interest in the topic prompted him to conduct experiments that went against the conventional belief that the dental tubules were filled with a vitreous like fluid and movement of the fluid caused pain. Since the tubules were believed to be void of nerves, the hypothesis did not hold up. His first experiment involved preparing a cylindrical cavity into dentin with a vacuum hose attached. Upon microscopic examination, he discovered that odontogenic projections along with their nucleus were sucked up into the tubule causing pain that lasted as long as the vacuum was on [7].

After several experiments involving different means of varying pressure within the dental tubule including an air stream, temperature changes, potassium chloride, and blotting paper, microscopic examination correlated distortion of odontoblastic processes within the tubules with dentinal pain. This pain is of short duration and wanes soon after the challenge is removed.

It should be noted that his hypothesis applies only to dentin and not to the integument of the pulp. When a healthy tooth is tested with heat or cold placed on enamel, the sensation felt is from dentin. Once caries has destroyed the dentin, the hydrodynamic effect no longer applies. By this time, an inflammatory response has begun in the pulp proper, and the pain threshold of the sensory nerves is reduced. The a-∂ fibers in the pulp are the first to respond with a sharp lancinating pain followed by an aching pain from the C-fibers. If the aching pain resolves quickly and there has not been a history of spontaneous pain, a pulp cap may be attempted. Any history of the patient having to take an analgesic for an ache from the suspect tooth precludes a conservative approach and calls for root canal treatment or extraction.

6.8 Electric Pulp Tester: (EPT)

Contrary to the designation of pulp tester, the EPT does not determine the health status of a pulp.

1. *What Does an Electric Pulp Tester (EPT) Do?*
   (a) Confirms continuity of the contents within the pulp chamber (It can indicate vitality, but not the health of the pulp. It is subject to misinterpretation.)
   (b) It should not be used as an alternative to a thermal test; rather, it is an adjunct to help interpret questionable results.
   (c) A "shock" is felt once the electric charge delivered reaches the stimulation threshold.
2. *How Does the EPT Work?*
   (a) The EPT sends an electric charge (Power) through a tooth intended to evaluate the status of a dental pulp. The presumption is that if a shock is felt, the pulp is vital. If it is not felt, the pulp is not vital. This is a fallacious assumption in that the EPT is merely a continuity tester.
3. *If the Pulp Is Not Vital, How Is the Circuit Completed and the EPT Digital Readout Turned On?*
   There are 2 paths electric current can follow when testing teeth.
   (a) The initial path involves a low power charge that traverses the surface of the entire root attachment to the PDL. Once the circuit is completed a digital readout will appear. The appearance of the readout confirms the circuit is completed even though the pulp chamber is void of a conduction medium (pulp tissue, blood, pus, etc.).
   (b) Once this initial path is completed, the voltage increases incrementally so long as the circuit is not broken. If it is broken the device will reset to avoid delivering a shock.
   (c) The rate voltage increases is controlled by a rotating dial that should be set at (~6) allowing the patient to interrupt the circuit in a timely fashion once the electric charge reaches the stimulation threshold and they feel a pulsing "Shock".
   (d) If the pulp canal is void of a conductive substance (i.e., pulp tissue), the max Power of the EPT cannot send a flow of current through the apex to viable tissue, thus a shock is not felt even when the output reaches its maximum.
4. *Why Isn't the Shock Felt as the Charge Traverses the PDL?*
   This failure to feel the shock is explained in the following discussion on "current density".
   (a) The answer lies in appreciation for the Power of the electric charge.
   (b)
   $$\text{Power} = \text{Amps} \times \text{Volts}. \quad P = I \times V$$
   (c) Power must reach or exceed the Sensory Threshold to be felt. Think about a 1.5 V battery on the tongue…Vs… a 9 V battery…Voila! "Sensory Threshold" exceeded!

5. *What Does the Digital Readings Mean?*

   The digital readout is an ordinal scale and is not a direct correlation to the actual power being delivered. Comparing readouts between teeth to determine the status of the pulp is flawed since the overall resistance of each circuit (that determines the magnitude of the electric charge applied) is not the same.

6. *Why Does a Patient Respond to the Power (P) of the Electric Charge (EC) When It Passes through the Pulp Chamber and Out the Apex but not Felt as It Passes from the Root through the PDL?*

   In order to understand this, let's review some basic electric theories where:
   Voltage (V) is the force that drives current.
   Current (I) is a defined measure of electrons, expressed in Amperes.
   Resistance (R) impedes the flow of electrons, expressed in Ohms.
   Power (P) is a measure of electrical energy.

$$\text{Volts} = \text{Amperes x's Resistance} \quad \mathbf{V} = \mathbf{I} \times \mathbf{R}$$

$$\text{Power} = \text{Volts x's Amperes} \quad \mathbf{P} = \mathbf{V} \times \mathbf{I}$$

7. *Why Is the Digital Reading for Anterior Teeth Usually Less Than for Molars?*

   First and foremost, recall the EPT digital readings are an ordinal scale and not a direct correlation to the actual voltage or current density.

   Resistance (R) inversely correlates to the overall area of the pathway just like small openings resist the flow of water through a pipe and large areas allow for water to flow readily.

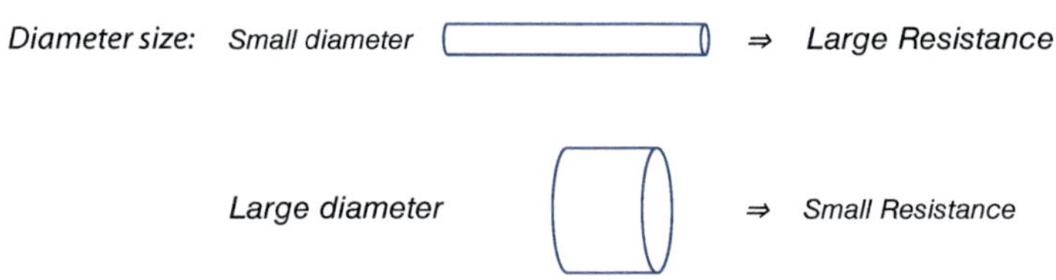

Simply put,

   (a) Very little force is required to get 10 gallons of water per minute to flow through a pipe with a 1 ft. diameter.
   (b) Now get that same 10 gallons per minute to flow through a pipe with a diameter of 1 inch.
   (c) Obviously, more force is required to overcome the resistance attributable to the smaller pipe.

8. Assuming this analogy is valid, the force (Voltage) required to drive current through a small area is considerably higher than through a large area. This leads one to conclude that a higher voltage is needed to stimulate single rooted anterior teeth than multi-rooted posterior teeth. Anterior teeth, however, usually respond at a lower ordinal number and theoretically a lower voltage. Thus, this

analogy is inadequate to explain why posterior teeth with multiple apexes respond at a higher reading than anterior single rooted teeth.

9. It is not just the voltage rather the Power (I × V) that results in the "shock" bringing into account the concept of "Current Density".
10. Current density "**J**" is defined as the amount of electric charge per unit time that flows through a given unit area (ua). An ampere is one coulomb of charge (6.24 x 10^{18} charge carriers) going past a given "ua" in one second.
    (a) *Where* **J** = **I/A²**
        J = current density.
        I = current flowing through the conductor in Amps/sec.
        A = cross-sectional unit area² in meters.

$$\text{Current Density} = \frac{\text{amount of electric charge (Amperes)}}{\text{Unit area in meters}^2}$$

    or CD = Amps ÷ ua²
    (b) ↑ Area = ↓ Current Density and a ↓ Resistance
    (c) ↓ Area = ↑ Current Density and an ↑ Resistance
    (d) Think of current as a group of electrons moving through a circuit at a given moment (like the 10 gallons of water), the larger area requires less voltage (force) to drive the electrons through the area resulting in less power. Once the power falls below the sensory threshold, pain is not felt. *Consequently, voltage must increase to increase the Power sufficiently to meet the Sensory Threshold***.** And this now accounts for multi-rooted teeth and teeth with open apexes to respond at a higher reading or possibly not at all if the apex is wide open.
    (e) Summary: As Current Density decreases the available amps per unit area also decreases. As the area of the apex increases, Voltage must also increase in order to maintain sufficient power to reach the Sensory Threshold.
11. *How Does This Relate to a Tooth?*
    (a) Keep in mind the 1.5 vs 9-volt battery. Also recall the reading from the digital readout is merely an ordinal scale does not represent the actual voltage generated. And the electric charge (Power = Volts x's Amps).
    (b) Teeth with small apexes have a higher current density (more amps per unit area) at a given voltage and therefore have sufficient power to reach the sensory threshold at a lower voltage.
    (c) Teeth with multiple apexes have an overall larger area and thus a lower current density (fewer amps per unit area) thus a higher voltage is needed to achieve sufficient power to reach the sensory threshold.
    (d) This is especially true of deciduous teeth and newly erupted teeth with open apexes. In fact, the current density (J) may be so low that the sensory threshold is not reached.
    (e) Note: the formula **J** = **I/Area²**… as the cross-sectional area increases the current density decreases exponentially.
12. A real-life experience illustrates this process well. Consider a cool dry day where static electricity has struck each time you reached for a doorknob. If you

were to approach the knob with just your fingertip you would be likely to experience a spark as the static electricity discharges from the tip of your finger to the knob. This would represent a high current density. On the other hand, if you were to grab the knob with the palm of your hand, you would most likely not experience a shock. The reason is that less voltage would be needed to allow the transfer of electrons since the larger area presents a lower current density **(J).** Lower amps/area^2 results in a lower power electric charge. $P = I \times V$ and a failure to reach the stimulation threshold.

References

1. Deshpande A, Verma S, Macwan C. Allergic reaction associated with the use of Eugenol containing dental cement in a young child. Aust J Dent. 2014;1(2):1007. ISSN:2381-9189.
2. Agnihotry A, Thompson W, Fedorowicz Z, van Zuuren EJ, Sprakel J. Antibiotic use for irreversible pulpitis. Cochrane Database Syst Rev. 2019;5(5):CD004969. https://doi.org/10.1002/14651858.CD004969.pub5. PMID: 31145805; PMCID: PMC6542501.
3. Lado EA, Richmond AF, Marks RG. Reliability and validity of a digital pulp tester as a test standard for measuring sensory perception. J Endod. 1988;14(7):352–6. https://doi.org/10.1016/S0099-2399(88)80197-3.
4. Abebe W. Review of herbal medications with the potential to cause bleeding: dental implications, and risk prediction and prevention avenues. EPMA J. 2019;10(1):51–64. https://doi.org/10.1007/s13167-018-0158-2. PMID: 30984314; PMCID: PMC6459456.
5. Fomete B, Saheeb BD, Obiadazie AC. A prospective clinical evaluation of the effects of chlorhexidine, warm saline mouth washes and microbial growth on intraoral sutures. J Maxillofac Oral Surg. 2015;14(2):448–53. https://doi.org/10.1007/s12663-014-0666-0. Epub 2014 Aug 15. PMID: 26028872; PMCID: PMC4444729.
6. Tolstunov L. Influence of immediate post-extraction socket irrigation on development of alveolar osteitis after mandibular third molar removal: a prospective split-mouth study, preliminary report. Br Dent J. 2012;213(12):597–601. https://doi.org/10.1038/sj.bdj.2012.1134. PMID: 23257808
7. Brännström M. Sensitivity of dentine. Oral Surg Oral Med Oral Pathol. 1966;21(4):517–26 . ISSN 0030-4220. https://doi.org/10.1016/0030-4220(66)90411-7.

Correction to: Pathway to Diagnosis and Management of Toothaches

Correction to:
E. Lado, R. Caudle, *Pathway to Diagnosis and Management of Toothaches*, https://doi.org/10.1007/978-3-031-75262-9

This book was inadvertently published with many errors and they have been corrected.

The updated versions of this book can be found at
https://doi.org/10.1007/978-3-031-75262-9

E. Lado, R. Caudle, *Pathway to Diagnosis and Management of Toothaches*,
https://doi.org/10.1007/978-3-031-75262-9_7

MAP of Dental Diagnosis

E. Lado, R. Caudle, *Pathway to Diagnosis and Management of Toothaches*,
https://doi.org/10.1007/978-3-031-75262-9

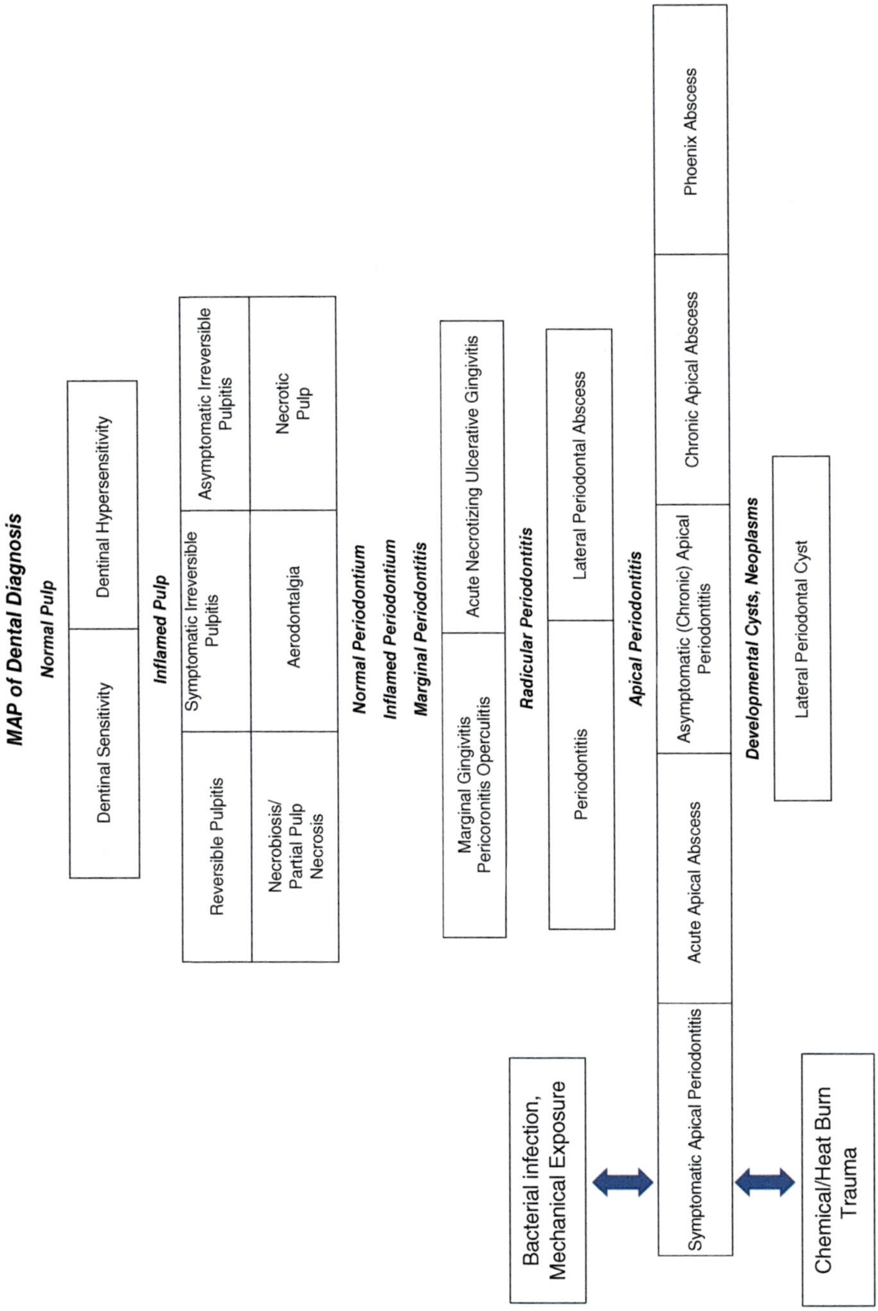
MAP of Dental Diagnosis
Normal Pulp
Dentinal Sensitivity
Dentinal Hypersensitivity
Inflamed Pulp
Reversible Pulpitis
Symptomatic Irreversible Pulpitis
Asymptomatic Irreversible Pulpitis
Necrobiosis/ Partial Pulp Necrosis
Aerodontalgia
Necrotic Pulp
Normal Periodontium
Inflamed Periodontium
Marginal Periodontitis
Marginal Gingivitis Pericoronitis Operculitis
Acute Necrotizing Ulcerative Gingivitis
Radicular Periodontitis
Periodontitis
Lateral Periodontal Abscess
Apical Periodontitis
Symptomatic Apical Periodontitis
Acute Apical Abscess
Asymptomatic (Chronic) Apical Periodontitis
Chronic Apical Abscess
Phoenix Abscess
Developmental Cysts, Neoplasms
Lateral Periodontal Cyst
Bacterial infection, Mechanical Exposure
Chemical/Heat Burn Trauma

Summary of Common Odontogenic Conditions

Normal Pulp

Attributes, Speculations, and Suggestions

- A normal pulp presents without any painful responses to everyday challenges.
- A pulp chamber protected by reparative dentin may not respond to thermal challenges simply because the change is temperature insufficient to trigger a neural response. In some teeth, the thickness of dentin is sufficient to block the flow of an electric charge from an electric pulp tester. In the absence of pain or abnormal radiographic findings, this condition does not require treatment.

Dentinal Sensitivity (DS)

Attributes, Speculations, and Suggestions

- Excellent discussions on dentinal sensitivity are published exploring the various causes and mechanism for dentinal sensitivity [1]. Presently the most favored theory is the hydrodynamic theory of dentinal pain proposed by Brännström.
- Dentin is comprised of tubules housing odontoblast processes, many accompanied by a-∂ nerve fibers. It is normally non-symptomatic UNLESS the dentinal tubule is open to the oral environment.
- These tubules are normally protected with a cover of enamel, cementum, or mineral deposits. Exposing unprotected tubules results in a sharp short duration pain to most challenges (thermal, chemical, mechanical, osmotic, desiccation). Dentinal sensitivity pain requires a stimulus and does not occur spontaneously. This pain is simply a warning signal that something is not right and needs attention.
- This pain is consistent with Brännström's Hydrodynamic theory of pain.

E. Lado, R. Caudle, *Pathway to Diagnosis and Management of Toothaches*,
https://doi.org/10.1007/978-3-031-75262-9

Dentinal Hypersensitivity (DH)

Attributes, Speculations, and Suggestions

- It has been suggested that prolonged exposure of the open dentinal tubules to various challenges results in injury to the odontoblastic processes resulting in an exaggerated painful response (Allodynia). This science is not settled but it is agreed that for sensitivity to occur the dentinal tubules must be open.
- However, we should recognize that most hypersensitivity arises from the root area as opposed to the coronal dentin. It has been proposed that the straight shape (not "S" shaped) and their greater diameter provide a greater opportunity for bacteria and toxins to penetrate and initiate an inflammatory process in the underlying pulp.
- Davari AR, and Porto IC, point out a number of etiologic factors as well as means of preventing and managing DH [2, 3].
- The solution requires either sealing the tubules or walling off the tubule from the pulp with reparative dentin.
- Dentinal pain MUST NOT BE CONFUSED with pulp pain arising from a pulp.
- Note: bleaching, tarter control toothpastes, acid etching, acid reflux, sweets, including sugar substitutes, smokeless tobacco, etc., will promote acid-producing bacteria that will disrupt the protective cover over dentin. Unless the reparative dentin is formed, the repeated insults may provoke an "allodynia."
- A possibility is that obliteration of the odontoblasts in cervical dentin results in micro pulp exposures that allow bacteria into the pulp canal and initiate an inflammatory response producing PgE_2 thereby lowering the pain threshold of the a-∂ fibers resulting in allodynia.

Inflamed Pulp

Attributes, Speculations, and Suggestions

- A diseased pulp can present with a variety of symptoms and responses to challenges.
- The symptoms and responses to test challenges reflect the status of the pulp. Once the pulp is invaded by bacteria or chemical/mechanical injury results in cell lysis, the disease process begins and is unlikely to be reversed. In rare instances pulps may recover by isolating healthy tissue from diseased tissue with a dentinal bridge. This rarely occurs in erupted teeth with fully formed root apex. Teeth with open apexes have a better chance of recovery because of the increased blood supply.

- The tell tail sign that the tooth is beyond self-repair is a history of spontaneous pulp pain. It should be noted that in some instances pulps will necrose with a minimum of spontaneous pain. The following conditions are stages expressed by a dying pulp.

Reversible Pulpitis

Attributes, Speculations, and Suggestions

- Reversible pulpitis is the body's response to injury involving the vital structures of the tooth. Since the dentinal tubules are in direct communication with the vital pulp tissue any challenge affecting the odontoblasts is perceived by the pulp as an attack of itself. As such, inflammatory mediators will be released even in the absence of an infection.
- Whenever the cell membranes are disrupted, PgE_2 is formed and the pain threshold of the a-∂ and C fibers is lowered resulting in a hyper response to a challenge. So long as the pain is elicited and NOT spontaneous it is presumed that removal of the challenge will allow the pulp to return to normal and possibly form tertiary dentin to further protect the pulp.

Symptomatic Irreversible Pulpitis

Attributes, Speculations, and Suggestions

- If the challenge is not removed, cells continue to lyse, and PgE_2 levels continue to rise so high that aching pain from C-fibers (found deeper within the pulp) becomes "SPONTANEOUS". The sharp shooting pain may still be provoked by thermal challenge, but the involvement of the C fibers will result in an underlying continuous dull aching pain.
- This patient will likely seek relief by applying OTC tooth remedies such as Benzocaine or eugenol-based products to the area or taking OTC analgesics. These OTC remedies can skew diagnostic tests.

Asymptomatic Irreversible Pulpitis

Attributes, Speculations, and Suggestions

- This condition is suggestive of pulp injury that causes cellular death (lysis) and is highly unlikely to respond positively to a pulp cap procedure. Recently erupted teeth with open apices may respond with formation of a dentinal bridge upon removal of the dying pulp and placement of calcium hydroxide on viable pulp tissue. If there is no involvement of the apical tissues this procedure may allow for completion of the root formation and provide a better support for a post and crown restoration.

- Once the apex has closed, pulp capping is not likely to be successful because the blood supply to the remaining pulp will not be sufficient to maintain vitality.

Partial Pulp Necrosis

Attributes, Speculations, and Suggestions

- Once the pulp tissues necrose a dead air space occupies the void and this often accounts for a specious interpretation of pulp testing. Thermal testing and electric pulp testing are nullified by a failure of the challenge to reach viable pulp tissue. It is not unusual for a patient to complain about excruciating pain upon eating ice cream yet unable to feel the application of cold on tooth structure. Invariably instrumentation of the pulp canal will provoke an intense painful response. By this stage significant levels of inflammatory mediators especially PgE_2 should be exiting the apex. A continuous aching pain will likely be accompanied by a sensitivity to apically directed forces including mastication and percussion. This condition may manifest as an aerodontalgia if the void within the canal is sealed.

Aerodontalgia

Attributes, Speculations, and Suggestions

- As previously described, Aerodontalgia results from air trapped within the pulp canal that is sealed coronally with a restoration and by viable, albeit diseased, remaining pulp at the apex. Application of "Charles Gas Law" that states increased temperature causes a gas to expand and when confined in a closed space pressure rises. Please review section on aerodontalgia. Pages 19 and 94 of the text.

Necrotic Pulp

Attributes, Speculations, and Suggestions

- This process of necrosis may start at the coronal part of the pulp from caries or apically from a blow severing the blood supply to the pulp. It is contingent on the complete necrosis of the remaining pulp in the chamber and canal. Unless the conditions for an aerodontalgia are present the pulp should not respond to any challenge. However, it should be noted that the void within the canal provides an ideal environment for the colonialization of microorganisms.

- *The condition often manifests as a discolored tooth with a history of trauma that occurred years previously but never hurt after it initially healed. Since there was no blood flow into the area there was no antimicrobial action. Little to no cell lysis occurred during this period so the presence of inflammatory mediators especially PgE_2 was nil and the tooth remained asymptomatic.*
- *It is presumed that a flair-up was due to pathogens finding their way to this ideal place* via *anachoresis. (Exemplified by an endocarditis caused by dental treatment).*

Normal Periodontium

Attributes, Speculations, and Suggestions

- Normal periodontium should be pink (genetic pigmentation exception) and comprised of three segments. The attached gingiva, periodontal ligament, and the col
- The col is a depression in the interdental papilla and is lined with epithelium of developmental origin comprised of the epithelium lining the tooth bud and the oral epithelium. This tissue is unique and forms the interdental papilla. Once the papilla is destroyed the epithelium is replaced by un-keratinized cells. A study on 20 young rhesus monkeys "concluded that the histological features and turnover-rate of epithelium in the interdental region are closely analogous to those of epithelium on other aspects of the teeth." but it did not define "closely analogous [4]."
- A search of Pub Med was not fruitful. Years ago, I was taught that the col (being unique) helped protect against periodontal disease but that once destroyed the area was no longer protective. I believe this would be an area worth exploring with the advances made in microbiology and immunity.
- I suspect ANUG may also render the interdental papilla region vulnerable to periodontal disease.
- Proper interdental cleaning and elimination of food impaction area are critical to preventing pocket formation along with known micro-flora.
- Proper use of a water irrigating device and interdental brushes could help maintain healthy interdental papilla.
- Normal periodontium does not bleed, stink, nor have a metallic taste to the exudate. Any of these symptoms should prompt a visit to the dentist.
- Dry mouth is a nemesis to the periodontium. Use of a mouth wetting agent is paramount. In the past lemon drops and other salivary promoters were used but most all contributed to root caries. Glycerin-based products are readily available and for patient with Schogren's disease or taking medications that cause dry mouth are very helpful. Saliva is protective against both caries and periodontal disease.

Inflamed Periodontium

Attributes, Speculations, and Suggestions

- Periodontitis is the progression of gingivitis apically into the attachment mechanism. Crestal bone is lost along with formation of a periodontal pocket as the gingival attachment moves apically.
- Pain is two-fold. First there will be periodontal pain associated with the C-fibers dominating the PDL along with infection brought on by food and bacteria accumulating in the pockets.
- The second pain is Sharp in quality from odontoblasts and a-∂ fibers located in the exposed dentinal tubules.
- Thus, it is possible for a periodontal lesion to present symptoms suggestive of dentinal sensitivity and/or hypersensitivity.
- There are several conditions other than apical that result in inflammation of the periodontium. I have divided them into 3 areas. The first is apical that has been discussed. The remaining 2 are marginal and radicular in nature. Marginal gingivitis involves inflammation of the unattached gingiva and col (embryologic formation of the interdental papilla) and the radicular attachment area.

Marginal Periodontitis

Gingivitis

Attributes, Speculations, and Suggestions

- Gingivitis is an inflammatory response to oral bacteria incorporated in a biofilm (known as plaque that is attached to tooth. It is easily removed with proper brushing but if allowed to remain in place for several days it will harden and require professional removal.
- Symptoms include some discomfort, an itchy or tingling feeling from the gums. Cardinal signs include inflammation of the gums, including a red, puffy appearance and bleeding due to brushing or flossing. Patients will often complain of finding blood on their pillow upon waking.
- This inflammation is easily treated simply by physical removal. However, when left for an extended period the inflammation will affect the supporting bone. Otherwise known as periodontitis.
- Marginal periodontitis includes gingival infections associated with third molar eruption and is best resolved by removal of the opposing tooth as well as the involved third molar.

Acute Necrotizing Ulcerative Gingivitis

Attributes, Speculations, and Suggestions

- Although ANUG is not considered a typical periodontal condition it is included here as a possible differential in the diagnosis of tooth pain. Also known as Vincent's angina or trench mouth the etiology is usually secondary to an overgrowth of fusobacteria and *spirochete bacteria which are normally found in the oral cavity.*
- Symptoms include painful raw denuded gingiva, punched-out papilla, putrid breath, metallic taste, a general feeling of malaise, possible fever.
- It is proposed to be a consequence of stress although there appears to be some controversy in the literature. Years ago, I would see several cases in my practice especially around finals time. For the past 30 years I have noticed a marked decrease of cases except in protracted cases of HIV where the CD4 count is below 200.
- Although the condition may respond to penicillin or amoxicillin/metronidazole combination along with chlorhexidine gluconate oral rinse, I still encourage otherwise healthy patients to improve their nutrition, get rest, and take vitamin C, and B complex and periodic rinses with 0.12% chlorhexidine gluconate and periodic swishing with Gly-oxide®.
- Magic mouth rinse may be an alternative solution to relieve pain from ANUG. Do not mix Benadryl with a salicylate or aspirin-containing solution such as Pepto Bismol or Kaopectate if sensitive to aspirin or salicylates. Maalox, or Milk of Magnesia is an acceptable alternative. Be sure to follow manufactures warnings.
- Eating may be a problem due to the pain so a diet supplement drink such as Boost® Ensure® or any of the proprietary supplements may be helpful.

Radicular Periodontitis

Periodontitis

Attributes, Speculations, and Suggestions

- Periodontitis is thought to be the major cause of tooth loss and has been linked to various health problems including heart disease.
- This association with health problems is most likely attributed to the insidious nature of the disease. Rarely does periodontitis cause the severity of pain comparable to the dental pulp. As such the patient is rarely motivated to seek professional care and usually becomes aware of the problem when informed that the tooth cannot be restored even with RCT because of the extent of bone loss.

- If the patient is experiencing pain from a periodontal abscess from a deep pocket temporary relief may be provided by debriding the pocket. Long term solution requires elimination of the pocket of requiring surgery. Unfortunately, the disease and elimination of the pocket will leave root surface exposed and tubules open leading to dentinal hypersensitivity. Meticulous home care and desensitizing the root surface is essential.
- The best method of managing the problem is periodic visits to the dentist and attention to proper maintenance. Some patients have an immune deficiency that prevents arresting the disease. Unfortunately, these patients are doomed to removable prosthesis.

Lateral Periodontal Abscess

Attributes, Speculations, and Suggestions

- Lateral Periodontal Abscess: can be a tricky diagnosis. Presence of a sinus tract and swelling can mimic a draining apical abscess (Chronic Apical Abscess). This abscess is often caused by a tooth fracture extending to the PDL attachment. Another common cause of such an abscess is a nidus of calculus remaining following a deep periodontal scaling where reattachment of the periodontium occurs occlusal to trapped debris.
- It can also occur from a lateral accessory canal if the pulp is undergoing necroses. Treatment is causal-dependent often requiring drainage. Diagnosis is facilitated by tracing a sinus tract with a gutta-percha cone and confirming the terminal path with radiographic imaging. Restorability will be a major consideration as to the preferred treatment.

Apical Periodontitis

Attributes, Speculations, and Suggestions

- Diseased apex is usually an extension of pulp disease as the bacteria, their toxins, and inflammatory mediators pass through the apex into the apical PDL. Once this happens the pain threshold of the nerves found in the PDL decreases. Teeth supported by the socket transmit applied forces to the PDL.
- Percussing a tooth does not reveal the status of the pulp, rather pain upon percussion reveals the condition of the periodontium.
- Although an abscess results in the apical attachment and PDL properly performed RCT will allow for regeneration of attachment mechanism. Inadequately performed RCT may result in a recurrence of the Acut Apical abscess (AAA). This reoccurrence has been tagged "Phoenix Abscess."

Symptomatic Apical Periodontitis

Attributes, Speculations, and Suggestions

- This condition (SAP) may arise from either the spread of inflammatory mediators from an infected pulp, trauma from a blow, or pronounced occlusal forces resulting from clenching/bruxing as well as from inflammation associated with proximal structures such as the sinus.
- Death of the pulp from chemical exposure can also cause a SAP since cell membranes are lysed and arachidonic acid released that is then converted to PgE^{2}.
- Inflammatory mediators, especially PgE_2, may seep through the apex prior to the invasion of bacteria. The levels found are above normal but not nearly in the range found once the bacteria invade the PDL resulting in cellular lysis. This tooth will be sensitive to percussion but NOT to palpation and certainly not have a history of swelling. There may be a widening of the PDL at the apex due to the accumulation of fluids (edema) just as a bump on the forehead may arise from a blow. There is NO INFECTION present with this condition unless it is caused by bacteria/pathogens.
- If the source of inflammation is suspected to be from an infected pulp antibiotics may be helpful. On the other hand, if the inflammation is due to trauma (Bruxing) or a chemical burn, antibiotics would NOT be warranted.
- NOTE: Antibiotic are not warranted to treat a pulpitis without evidence of systemic involvement of pathogens unless they are immune compromised or uncontrolled diabetic with a pulpitis if systemic involvement (lymphadenitis, fever, malaise) is anticipated.

Acute Apical Abscess

Attributes, Speculations, and Suggestions

- Once bacteria enter the PDL through the apex marks the beginning of an apical abscess. It can take as long as 12 days for radiographic evidence to confirm bone resorption caused by the abscess.
- Absence of a Periapical radiolucency (PARL) is not pathognomonic. Radiographs depict a 2-dimensional image of a 3-dimensional condition and are at best helpful in diagnosis. A tooth presenting with a vestibular swelling may appear normal on imaging. This is commonly seen when there is fenestration of the apex through the bone and the abscess has pointed out of bone.
- Swelling is a common finding with an abscess but should not be the determinant finding since until the cortex is breached the abscess is confined to bone. Also, until the pus has egressed the periosteum the swelling will be hard and not fluctuant.
- The salient point defining an abscess is pain upon palpation. Levels of PgE_2 soar with an abscess due to the increased numbers of cells being lysed.

- With an increase of inflammatory mediators there is also a tendency to develop a cellulitis characterized by a broad area of swelling not confined to the area of the suspect tooth's root apex.
- Patients will often put a warm washcloth over the area. This is a NO, NO… by placing a warm compress externally there is a tendency to draw the infection to the surface having it "point" (drain) externally. This must be discouraged since external lesion is more difficult to manage. Cold compress is OK or warm saline rinses will help to draw the pus toward the vestibule where it is most likely to cause the least damage.

Asymptomatic (Chronic) Apical Periodontitis (AAP)

Attributes, Speculations, and Suggestions

- Asymptomatic Apical Periodontitis (AAP) as the name implies is without any symptoms. It is often seen in conjunction with a sterile necrotic pulp caused by trauma, failed pulp cap, or chemical burn, in which the pulp dies under sterile conditions or bacteria are being held in check by the bodies defense system.
- A large PARL (>2 mm) is characteristic of this condition. It is often discovered unexpectedly upon radiographic imaging. This condition is long standing with minimal levels of PgE_2 being produced. Therefore, there is little discomfort associated with it.
- Surprisingly, the painless condition often becomes very uncomfortable when endodontic treatment is initiated. This has been attributed to the presence of anaerobic bacteria in the lesion being exposed to O_2 dying and releasing endotoxins precipitating post-op pain.
- When accessing the canal for RCT advise the patient of the possible discomfort and suggest starting an NSAID if not contraindicated by the medical history. A script for an antibiotic may also be appropriate but taken only if symptoms arise.

Chronic Apical Abscess

Attributes, Speculations, and Suggestions

- This also is usually characterized by a large periapical radiolucency (PARL) (>2MM) and asymptomatic. Although pus periodically drains from the abscess, other than a periodic "Bad Taste," the condition is painless. Drainage usually occurs through a sinus track; an open pulp canal can provide for egress of pus.
- Since the lesion is open drainage allows inflammatory mediators (especially PgE_2) to escape, lowering the concentration and thus diminishing the effect of lowering the pain threshold of afferent nerves (a-∂ and C fibers).

- Although timely treatment should be provided this is not an emergent condition and antibiotic coverage is not needed unless the patient presents contributory "Risk Factors."
- Proper healing would include resolution of the sinus tract. Even though the treated area appears to heal. Follow-up imaging would be appropriate.

Phoenix Abscess

Attributes, Speculations, and Suggestions

- A Phoenix abscess presents the same as an Acute Apical Abscess EXCEPT imaging shows a large PARL that would have been considered an "asymptomatic apical periodontitis" (AAP) or a chronic apical abscess (CAA) if a sinus tract was present and closed off.
- It is often seen as an outcome of a failed pulp cap in which the pulp died quietly/ asymptomatically, and a follow-up evaluation never occurred.
- Had it been discovered prior to presenting with pain the condition would have presented conditions consistent with an AAP, or CAA. Both conditions are asymptomatic and found combined with a necrotic pulp.
- Therein lies the problem. The condition never caused pain (the main motivator to seek dental treatment.)
- The abscess became acute when bacteria found a void in the pulp canal that provided ideal conditions to propagate, lysing cell membranes, releasing arachidonic acid, that was then converted to PgE_2 along with all the other inflammatory mediators. Absence of a sinus tract allowed these mediators to concentrate and create all the conditions consistent with an AAA.
- The name Phoenix provides a likely scenario of the progression of the condition.
- A diagnostic consideration th*is* finding should provoke is to confirm the status of the pulp. A vital healthy pulp could suggest the lesion is neoplastic.

Developmental Cysts, Neoplasms

Lateral Periodontal Cyst

Attributes, Speculations, and Suggestions

- This is a cyst formed from odontogenic remnants including Hertwig's epithelial root sheath.
- They are defined as non-keratinized and non-inflammatory developmental cysts located adjacent or lateral to the root of a vital tooth. They rarely cause divergence of the roots and are usually asymptomatic. Being asymptomatic they are normally found by radiographic imaging.

Numerous Other Neoplasms

One needs to be cognizant of a multitude of neoplastic entities that may be found upon dental examination and prepared to refer the patient to a facility or practitioner capable of managing such conditions. Unfortunately, many conditions are with or without symptoms and therefore likely to spread possibly even becoming life threatening.

Table of Pain Descriptors

This table is provided to facilitate communication with a patient describing their pain.

E. Lado, R. Caudle, *Pathway to Diagnosis and Management of Toothaches*,
https://doi.org/10.1007/978-3-031-75262-9

This questionnaire may be used as a prompt to ensure pertinent information is not overlooked due to a misuse of words.

		Evaluative		
Intensity				
Mild		**Moderate**		**Severe**
Annoying	*Troublesome*	*Miserable*	*Intensive*	*Unbearable*
		Sensory		
Temporal				
Flickering	*Pulsing*	*Throbbing*	*Beating*	*Pounding*
Spatial				
Spreading	*Jumping*	*Radiating*	*Flashing*	*Shooting*
Punctate Pressure				
Pricking	*Boring*	*Drilling*	*Stabbing*	*Lancing*
Incisive Pressure				
	Sharp	*Cutting*	*Lancing*	
Constrictive Pressure				
Pinching	*Pressing*	*Gnawing*	*Cramping*	*Crushing*
Traction Pressure				
	Tugging	*Pulling*	*Wrenching*	
Thermal				
Warm	*Hot*	*Burning*	*Scalding*	*Searing*
Brightness				
Tickling	*Tingling*	*Itchy*	*Smarting*	*Stinging*
Dullness				
Dull	*Sore*	*Hurting*	*Aching*	*Heavy*
Miscellaneous				
Tender	*Taut*	*Rasping*	*Splitting*	*Tearing*
		Affective		
Tension				
Nagging	*Dragging*	*Tiring*	*Fatiguing*	*Exhausting*
Autonomic				
	Nauseating	*Sickening*	*Choaking*	*Suffocating*
Fear				
	Fearful	*Frightful*	*Dreadful*	*Terrifying*
Punishment				
Punishing	*Grueling*	*Cruel*	*Vicious*	*Killing*

Diagnostic Questionnaire Prompt

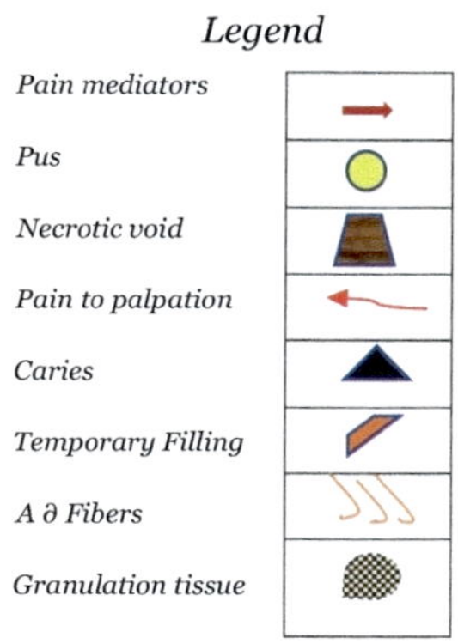

E. Lado, R. Caudle, *Pathway to Diagnosis and Management of Toothaches*,
https://doi.org/10.1007/978-3-031-75262-9

Schematic of Diagnostic "Snap Shots"

See Figs. 1, 2, 3, 4, 5, 6, 7, 8, 9, 10, 11.

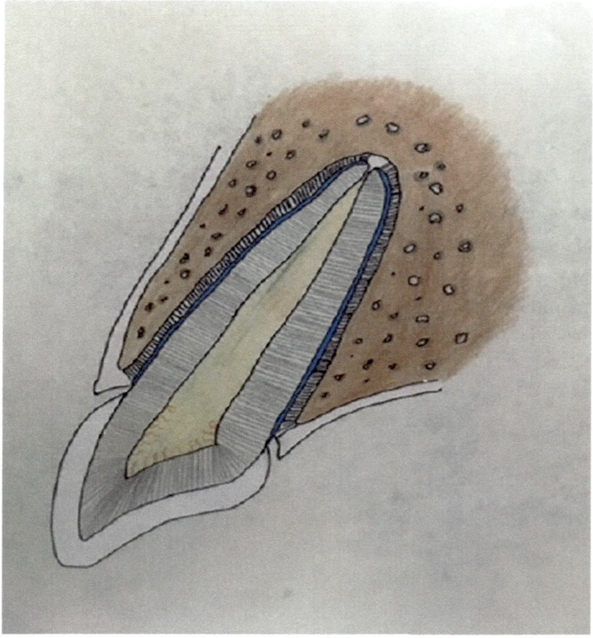

Fig. 1 Normal Pulp*. * *OLD TERMINOLOGY*

E. Lado, R. Caudle, *Pathway to Diagnosis and Management of Toothaches*, https://doi.org/10.1007/978-3-031-75262-9

Fig. 2 Symptomatic apical periodontitis (SAP). Acute apical periodontitis*. * *OLD TERMINOLOGY*

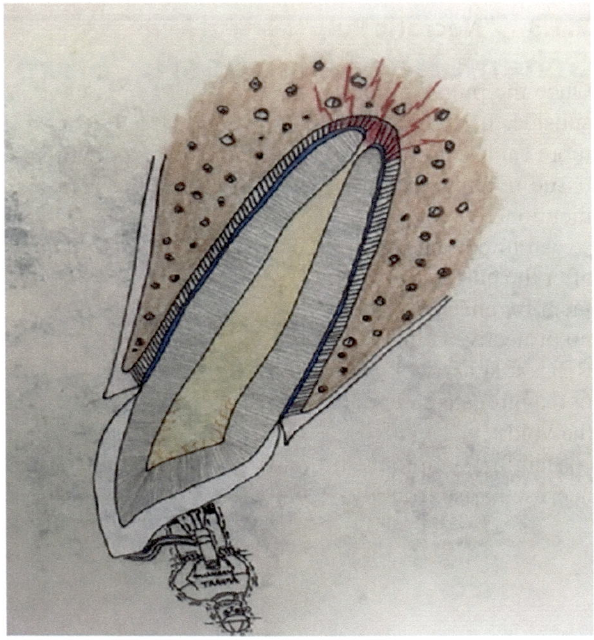

Fig. 3 Reversible pulpitis*(Allodynia?). * *OLD TERMINOLOGY*

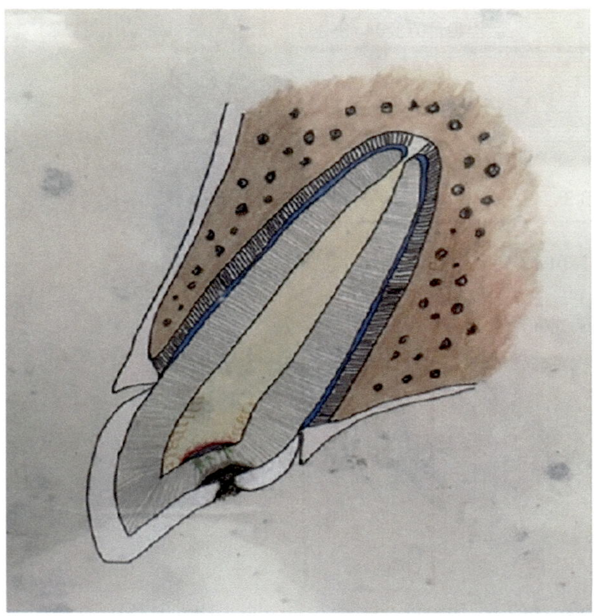

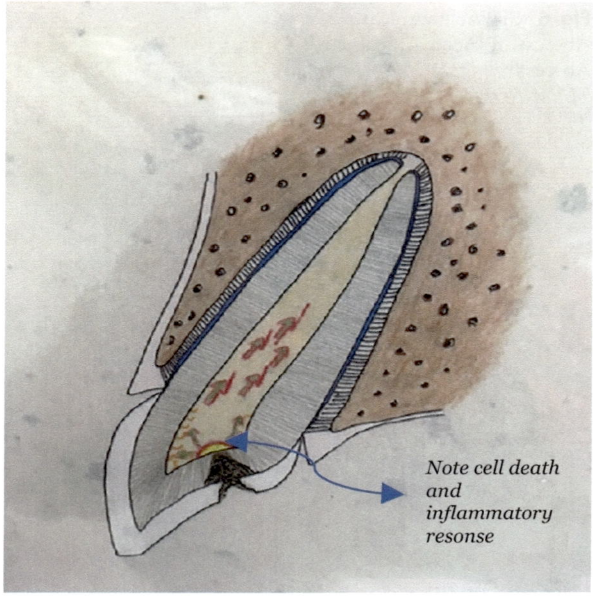

Fig. 4 Symptomatic Irreversible pulpitis (SIP) Irreversible pulpitis. (IP)*. * *OLD TERMINOLOGY*

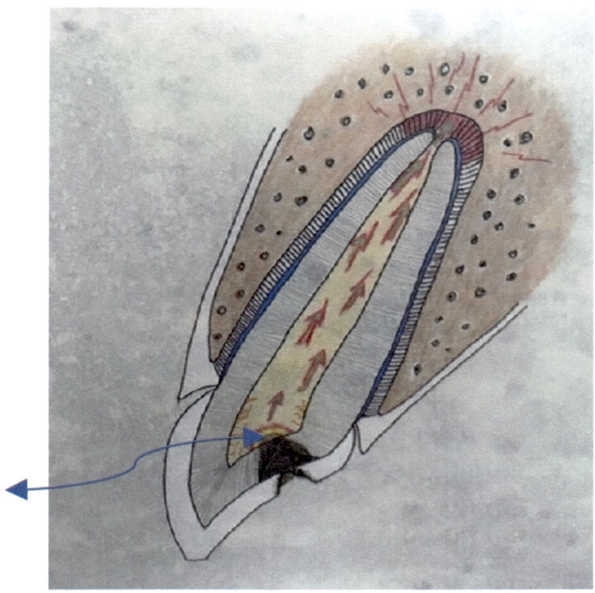

Fig. 5 SIP/SAP. IP/Acute Apical Periodontitis*. * *OLD TERMINOLOGY*

Fig. 6 SIP/Acute Apical Abscess. IP/Acute Apical Abscess*. * *OLD TERMINOLOGY*

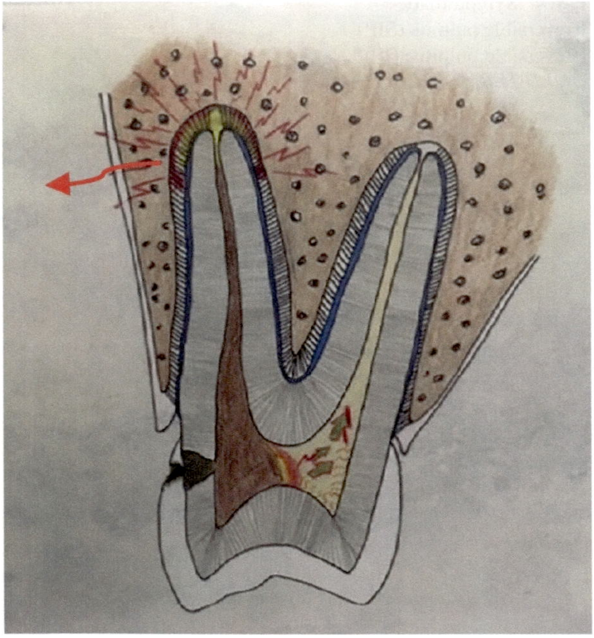

Fig. 7 Necrotic pulp/ Acute Apical Abscess. NP/ AAA*. * *OLD TERMINOLOGY*

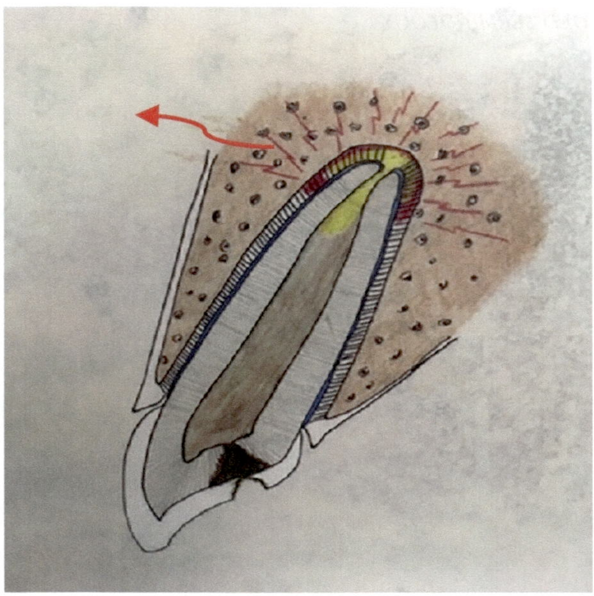

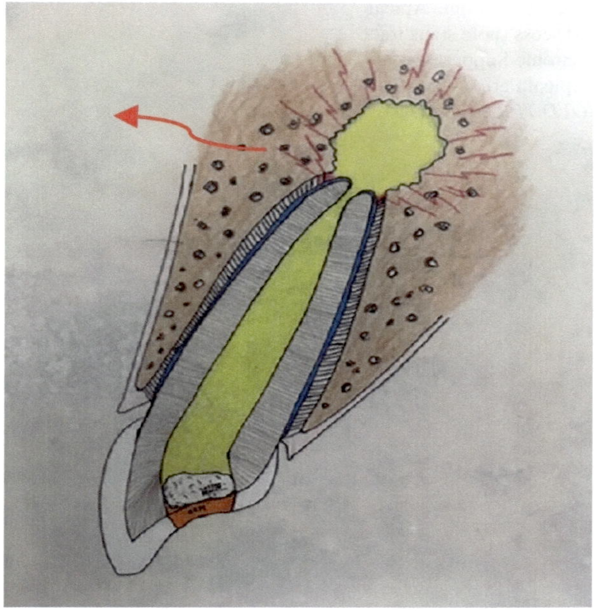

Fig. 8 Asymptomatic PARL becomes symptomatic. Phoenix Abscess*??? Necrotic pulp/AAA. Periapical radiolucency PARL. History of long standing PARL. * *OLD TERMINOLOGY*

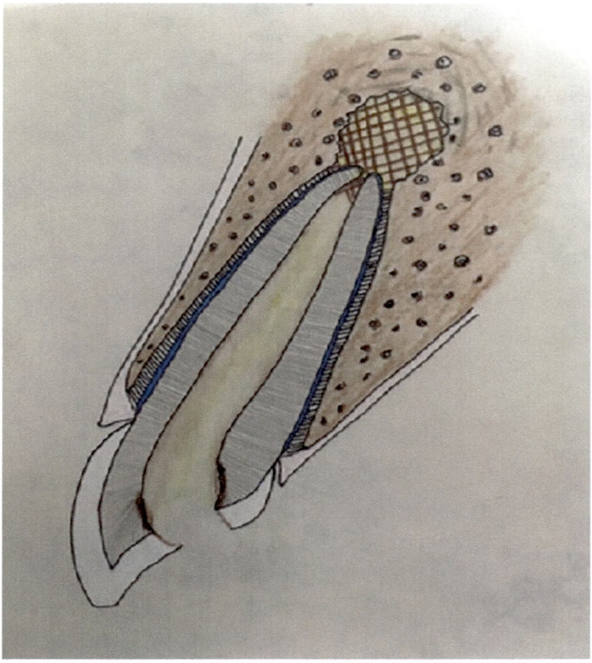

Fig. 9 Asymptomatic Apical Periodontitis. Chronic Apical Periodontitis* CAP*. * *OLD TERMINOLOGY*

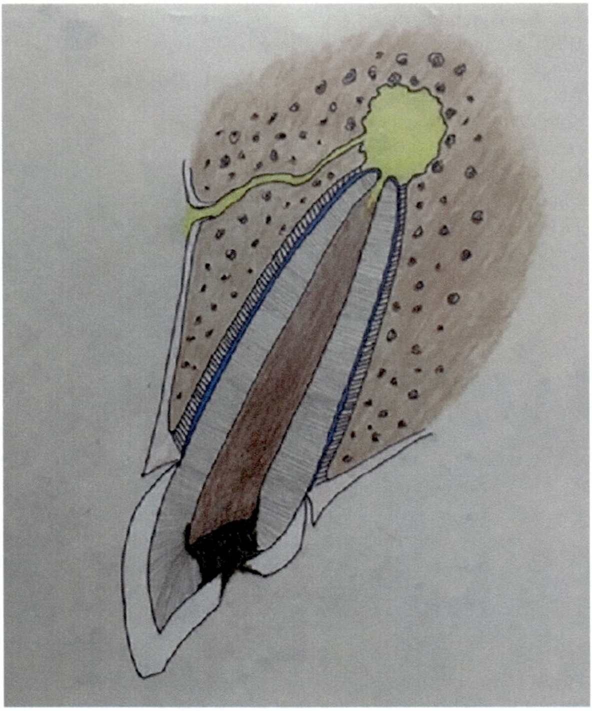

Fig. 10 Chronic Apical Abscess (note sinus tract. Chronic Suppurative Apical Periodontitis*). * *OLD TERMINOLOGY*

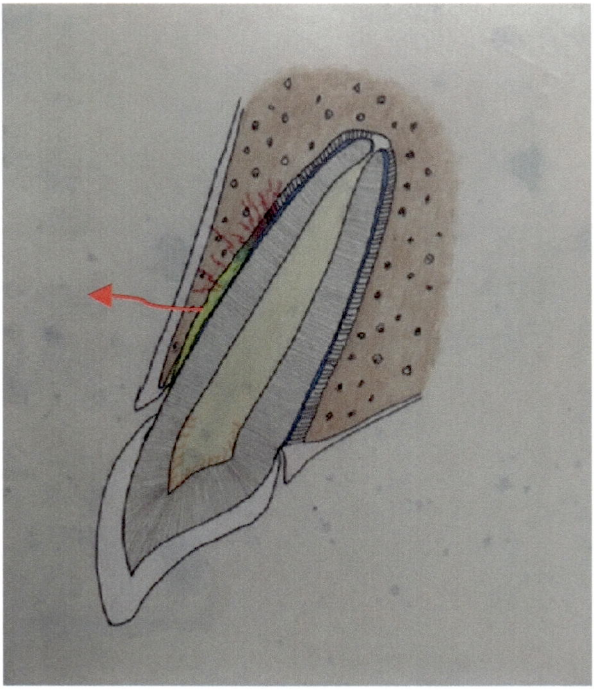

Fig. 11 Lateral Periodontal Abscess*. * *OLD TERMINOLOGY*

References

1. West N, Lussi A, Seong J, Hellwig. Dentin hypersensitivity: Pain mechanisms and aetiology of exposed cervical dentin. Clin Oral Investig. 2013;17(Suppl 1):S9–S19.
2. Davari AR, Ataei E, Assarzadeh H. Dentin Hypersensitivity: etiology, diagnosis and treatment; a literature review. J Dent Shiraz Univ Med Sci. 2013;14(3):136–45.
3. Porto IC, Andrade AK, Montes MA. Diagnosis and treatment of dentinal hypersensitivity. J Oral Sci. 2009;51(3):323–32.
4. McHugh WD. The interdental gingivae. J Periodontal Res. 1971;6(4):227–36.

GPSR Compliance

The European Union's (EU) General Product Safety Regulation (GPSR) is a set of rules that requires consumer products to be safe and our obligations to ensure this.

If you have any concerns about our products, you can contact us on ProductSafety@springernature.com

In case Publisher is established outside the EU, the EU authorized representative is:

Springer Nature Customer Service Center GmbH
Europaplatz 3
69115 Heidelberg, Germany

Batch number: 10732044

Printed by Printforce, the Netherlands